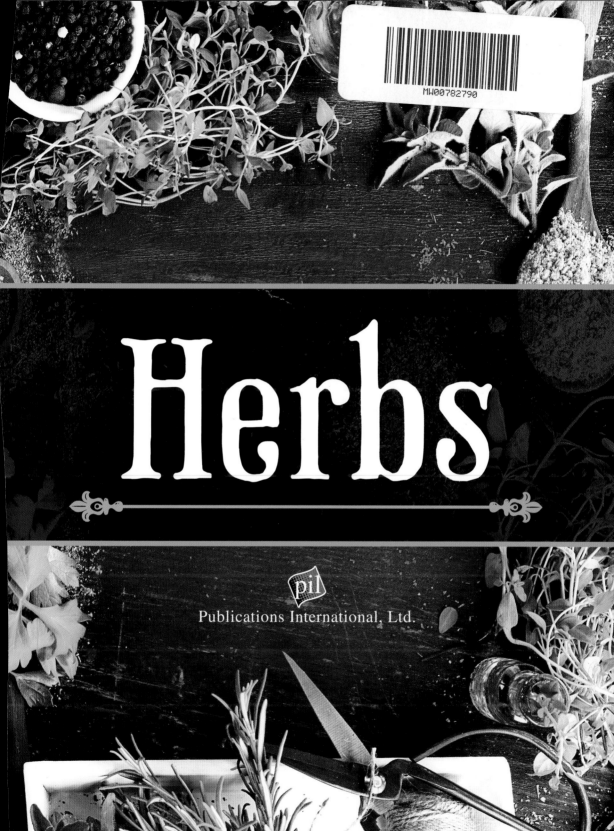

Herbs

pil

Publications International, Ltd.

Note: Neither the editors of Publications International, Ltd., nor the authors, consultants, editors, or publisher take responsibility for any possible consequence from any treatment, procedure, exercise, dietary modification, action, or application of medication or preparation by any person reading or following the information in this book. The publication of this book does not constitute the practice of medicine, and this book does not attempt to replace your physician or your pharmacist. Before undertaking any course of treatment, the authors, consultants, editors, and publisher advise the reader to check with a physician or other health care provider.

Contents

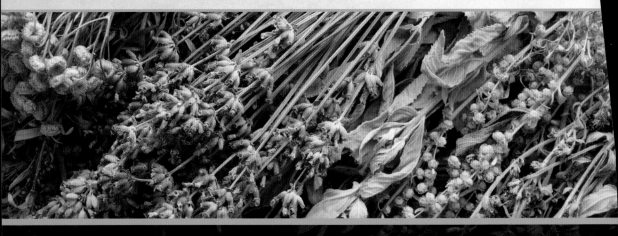

Introduction

Of the millions of plants that grace our world, herbs, by far, are the most useful and intriguing. For millennia, we have used herbs to flavor our foods, perfume our bodies and homes, decorate our environments, and cure our ills.

Their usefulness to human beings elevates even the most common roadside herbs to hallowed status. Take the dandelion, for instance—that ubiquitous invader of manicured lawns. How can we call this vital herb a weed when it provides us with nutritious salad greens, a delectable coffee substitute, a skin cleanser, and remedies for myriad ailments?

Herbs possess a natural grace and alluring beauty that sets them apart from other decorative garden plants. Our ancient ancestors recognized the value of herbs for their survival, using them as food, medicine, and even poison. Early in the Eastern world,

physicians wrote tomes on herbal remedies, some prized to this day as authoritative medical sources. Druids revered the oak and mistletoe, both rich in medicinal attributes. Later, the Greeks and Romans cultivated herbs for medicinal and culinary uses as well. Hippocrates, considered the father of Western medicine, prescribed scores of curative herbs and taught his students how to use them. In the Middle Ages, monks grew herbs in monastery gardens throughout Europe.

It was the search for precious herbs and spices that led Europeans to the New World. There they found scores of new plants which they brought back to the courts of England, Spain, and France. By the early 18th century, herb gardens were common throughout the continent. Colonists venturing to America brought herbs and seeds with them to cultivate in their new home.

The advent of the Industrial Revolution, however, spurred an exodus of people from rural to urban areas, and herbs gradually lost their mystique as science captured the imaginations of an increasingly sophisticated populace. Urban dwellers, with limited access to gardens, began to buy their medicines and foods instead of growing and preparing them at home.

But herbs enjoyed a renaissance as our technology-laden culture looked back to the benefits and charms of more natural times. Today, herb gardening and cultivation is an industry for some and a satisfying hobby for many others. As countless people are discovering, the use of herbs is as varied and intriguing as the breadth of their scents and foliage.

What exactly is an herb? No group of plants is more difficult to define. In general, an herb is a seed-producing plant that dies down at the end of the growing season and is noted for its aromatic and/or medicinal qualities. How did we decide which plants to include in this book? We chose those herbs that we judged the easiest to grow and the most useful for creating savory meals, aromatics, decorations, and herbal medicines.

Sooner or later, most herbal enthusiasts decide to try their hands at growing a few of their favorite herbs. We may start out with a single basil plant in a terra-cotta pot or window box. But once we start, we often find we cannot stop. That pot becomes a backyard garden, and that window box venture springboards into a lush, landscaped collection of fennel, garlic, and chives.

Most herbs thrive with very little care. These rugged, hardy plants survive and even flourish in poor soil and with wide temperature fluctuations that would prove disastrous for other cultivated species. A large part of herbs' appeal is their ability to respond well to their surroundings without excessive care.

Herbs fit beautifully into any landscape. Ground-hugging thyme is a perfect choice for planting between cracks in a flagstone walk. Tall clumps of angelica or rue provide attractive, dramatic accents in flower borders. Nasturtium, calendula, chives, and lavender add vibrant color to a garden and make handsome decorations as well. This book provides the basics on how to grow, propagate, harvest, and store the most popular herbs. It also includes advice on how to use herbs in your home and garden.

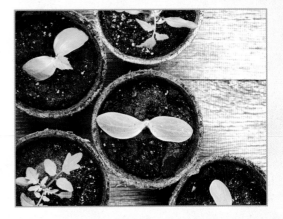

Cooks will find that an herb garden provides a tremendous opportunity for experimenting in the kitchen. The addition of just a teaspoon or two of a particular herb can transform an ordinary recipe into a gourmet feast. Whether you want to grow a few herbs in your kitchen window as a source of fresh flavoring for your meals, or you wish to design and plant an elaborate formal herb garden, you'll find here the basic information you need to get started. And as you become more familiar with herbs, you'll probably find yourself increasing the amount and varieties you grow.

Growing Herbs

If you're like most beginning gardeners, you may be put off by the prospect of growing herbs. Like children, herbs do require care and attention. But once you understand the basics of herb gardening, you'll soon be enjoying the delectable fruits of your labor. Begin by asking yourself how you plan to use your herbs. Do you like to cook? Then consider growing culinary standards such as parsley, rosemary, sage, and thyme. Will you make teas? Then plant mint, which comes in scores of varieties. If you intend to put your produce to cosmetic purposes, think of aloe, a wonderful skin refresher, or calendula, one of nature's most potent topical healers. For ornamental purposes, how about lavender or nasturium? Perhaps you'd like to try your hand at varied herbal crafts. Plant yarrow, hyssop, or santolina. Of course, you don't need one purpose to grow herbs—it's perfectly all right to mix and match. All you need to do is get started.

The key to success in growing an easy-care herb garden is to choose plants that thrive in the type of soil, water, and light available in your area. If you live in a part of the country with rich, moist soil and sunlight only part of the day, consider planting rue, sweet woodruff, peppermint, and spearmint. If your soil is dry, rocky, or sandy, grow sage, thyme, chamomile, and oregano, which thrive in those conditions. It's possible to live just about anywhere and produce an herb garden to enrich your senses and your pantry.

Of course, you're not restricted by your environment. If your area does not have the right conditions to support a particular herb, you can manipulate the soil, water, and nutrients to accommodate its needs. One of the simplest methods of growing herbs unsuited to your area is to plant them in containers. Another method is to fill a planting bed with the type of soil your plants require. To do this, remove the existing soil in the bed to a depth of 8 to 10 inches. Then replace the soil with a mix you've bought or prepared yourself. Because the level of your soil will be shallow, it's best to choose herbs that do not produce deep tap roots.

An alternative method is to construct a raised bed of the same depth. This works well if your plants require good drainage, or if the added height from a raised bed will give your herbs better visibility. You may enrich the soil of your beds by adding compost, lime, sand, or peat moss, depending on the particular needs of the herbs you choose.

Although light conditions are more difficult to control than soil conditions, you can adjust them to some extent. If you live in a sunny, hot area, look for ways to shade your plants. Perhaps you could construct a fence or simple arbor to provide a quick source of shade. For a long-term solution, plant leafy trees or hedges where you plan to grow herbs.

Soil Mix Recipes

These three basic soil mixes work well for most herbs. Note that these recipes are general guidelines. You may vary them somewhat without suffering disastrous results.

Sandy, well-drained mix

- 2 parts medium to coarse sand
- 1 part perlite
- 1 part potting soil or garden loam

Average soil mix

- 1 part potting soil or garden loam
- 1 part moistened peat moss or compost
- 1 part sand or perlite

Rich, moist mix

- 1 part potting soil or garden loam
- 1 part moistened peat moss or compost

If you don't get enough light, thin out adjacent trees and shrubs to let in more. Or you can plant your herbs in containers and shuttle them in and out of the sun. Most potted plants need to spend at least half a day in a sunny location; keep your containers small enough to rest on a wheeled base so you can move the herbs quickly and easily.

If you wish to grow herbs indoors, set plants under an artificial light source to ensure that they prosper. A few grow lamps can augment or replace existing natural light.

Beginning herb gardeners, eager to nurture their plants, often make the mistake of watering their gardens every day. Don't do this. Herbs need only about 1 inch of water a week. If your area gets very hot in the summer, if you have sandy soil, or if winds tend to dry out your garden, then you may need to water more often. But resist the urge to overwater. Not only does overwatering cause herbs to lose their flavor and fragrance, excess moisture may lead to fatal fungal diseases in plants.

The best way to begin a garden is to make a list of the plants you'd like to grow. Then note their soil, light, and water needs; height and spread; and any special details, such as foliage, flower color, or unusual growth habits. Make a secondary list of plants you might enjoy growing if you have room left in your garden. Sketch the garden area to scale (for example, 1 inch on the sketch represents 1 foot on the ground), decide on the size and shape of the planting beds, and determine where in the beds you will place each plant. Once you have filled in all your favorite plant varieties, choose from your secondary list to fill any empty spots. If you have planted perennials and are waiting for them to fill in the garden, you can plant annuals in the spaces the first year or two. Be sure to consider the natural features of your garden, including its topography and the presence of trees or shrubs. These factors influence the amount of light and water available to your herbs.

Growing Herbs Indoors

Of course, you don't need a backyard or even a patio to grow herbs. You can cultivate your garden indoors. Indoor gardens, in fact, have some advantages over outdoor gardens. Herbs in pretty containers enhance any decor and often create dramatic design effects when used as centerpieces or bookends. What better place for culinary herbs than a kitchen countertop? And nothing brightens a rainy day like a thriving indoor plant, providing you with a link to the great outdoors. While herbs grown indoors may not be as vigorous as those grown in a garden, it's possible to produce a more-than-adequate tabletop crop.

Herbs prefer at least four or five hours of strong sunlight every day. If it's not possible to give them sunlight, give your herbs eight to ten hours of artificial light daily. Try to maintain a constant temperature in the room that houses your plants. Like people, herbs dislike extreme fluctuations in temperature. Herbs also need good air circulation to minimize incidence of pests and disease.

Your indoor herbs also need adequate drainage. Use clay or plastic pots with holes covered with pebbles or newspaper. To complement your decor, place the containers in a trough or tray of ceramic, wicker, or tin. If you plant herbs in a decorative jar that has no water holes, place a layer of gravel or pebbles on the bottom, followed by a thin layer of broken charcoal to "sweeten" the soil, or keep it clean of pests and disease. Following these procedures allows soil to drain and prevents waterlogging.

In any case, don't use soil from your yard. It may contain disease organisms and pests that could flourish in a warmer indoor environment. Instead, buy a soil mix, or make one of sterilized loam combined with sand. Compost—either purchased or made from scratch—works well, too. Many of the most common garden herbs found in this book prefer a neutral soil. A pH between 6 and 7.5 is optimum, but most will adjust from a pH of 5 to 8. (A pH of 7 is neutral. A higher number indicates alkaline soil and a lower number designates acidic soil.) Compost alone helps adjust the soil's pH. If your soil tends to be acidic, you can make it more neutral by adding lime to the soil mix or compost. To make soil more acidic, add peat moss. Your local nursery should also have specific suggestions on how to improve the soil conditions where you live.

Most herbs do not require much in the way of fertilizer. In fact, if you feed them too much, they may look extra lush, but they can lose much of their flavor and even their medicinal properties. Your best bet is to mix compost into the ground and, if your soil is poor, use some fish emulsion and/or seaweed to fertilize it. Perennial herbs also appreciate a fish emulsion spray at least a few times a year. Water indoor herbs only when the top inch or so of soil has dried out. Your watering needs will vary according to the temperature and humidity of your room. If your house is centrally heated and kept at a fairly high temperature, you may need to water every other day. Because indoor herbs are not as prolific as those grown out-of-doors, harvest your herbs with restraint.

Herbs Suited for Container Growth

Aloe	Geranium, scented	Marjoram	Rue
Basil	Ginger	Oregano	Sage
Calendula	Horsetail	Nasturtium	Savory, summer
Catnip	Lavender	Parsley	Spearmint
Cayenne pepper	Lemon balm	Peppermint	Thyme
Chives		Rosemary	

Where Do I Get My Plants

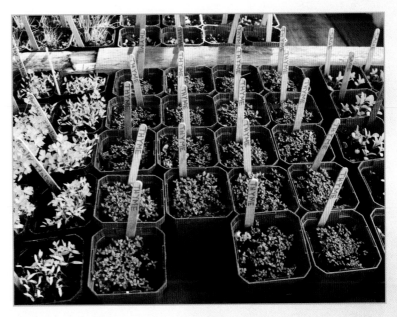

New plants come into being in five ways. A simple, inexpensive source is seeds. The best way to propagate most annuals is from seed. The second source of new plants is rooting cuttings from perennials. Many plant stems generate their own roots if you cut them from a parent plant and insert them into a growing mixture. A third method of getting new plants is through layering. Most perennial herbs with sprawling stems layer well. Press a stem into the ground and mound dirt over it. When a root has formed, cut the stem from the mother plant and repot it. Another easy and inexpensive way to acquire new plants is through division. You simply pull apart the roots of a large perennial plant to create several smaller ones. Choose plants with roots that sprout from the base and have more than one stalk. Finally, you can purchase plants from a nursery or garden shop. If you're not on a budget, this is the quickest and easiest way to obtain an established herb planting.

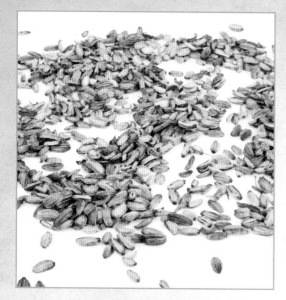

Seeds: You can start plants from seed in two ways: Sow the seeds directly in their garden bed, or start them in containers and transplant them later. How you start your seeds depends on the type of herb you wish to grow. Some herbs—especially annuals—grow quickly from seed, so they can be sown easily in their permanent locations. These include basil, calendula, chamomile, chives, and nasturtium. Other herbs don't like to be transplanted. For that reason, they, too, are easier to grow directly in beds. These include angelica, anise, borage, caraway, chervil, coriander, and dill. Still other herbs—lavender, marjoram, rosemary, and rue, for example—are slow starters or difficult to germinate. Thus, it is wise to start them indoors in containers and transplant them later.

Be sure to label your rows. Don't fool yourself into thinking you'll remember what's what. It's easy to forget by the time annuals come up—in about two weeks; perennials take two weeks or longer.

Cuttings: The best time to take cuttings of herbs is during the middle of the growing season, usually in late spring or early summer, before the herbs have flowered. Fill a container with a moist rooting medium. Your cuttings will live in this medium until they grow roots. At one time, coarse sand was the standard medium for rooting cuttings. Sand still works fine, but better alternatives are available, such as equal amounts of perlite mixed with peat moss and vermiculite. Or you can combine one part polymer soil additive (which has been expanded with water) and two parts peat moss.

With a sharp knife, cut a stem 3 to 6 inches long from the parent plant. Cut just below where the leaf attaches to the stem. Be careful not to crush the cutting. Carefully remove all leaves and shoots from the bottom one-half to two-thirds of the cutting: A tear in the stem can become a site for rot. Try to transplant your cuttings within 15 to 20 minutes. If that's not possible, place cuttings in water and replant as soon as you can. Poke a hole in your potting medium and insert the cuttings. Don't crowd them

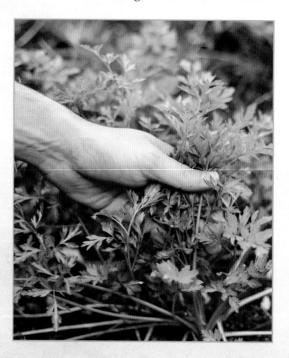

or you'll inhibit air circulation, which could encourage fungal growth. Water the cuttings immediately, but don't get water on the leaves. Keep the soil damp continuously. Place the cuttings in a spot that receives a generous amount of light, but don't put them in direct sunlight. After a week to ten days, check to see whether any roots have appeared. Do this by gently inserting a knife blade under the cutting and lifting it out. If you don't see any roots, reinsert the cutting and check it again in another week to ten days. Some plants take six or more weeks to root.

Once the roots are a quarter-inch long, plant the cutting in a small pot filled with commercial potting mix or one you've made. Water from above, and use a drip tray. Don't allow plants to stand in water for more than two hours. Keep the potted cutting out of direct sunlight for a week to avoid wilting the plant. Grow the cutting as a potted plant for a couple of months before transplanting it to the garden.

Layering is suitable for many perennials with strong stems. Select an outer stem from the base of the plant and push it to the earth. Mound a pile of dirt on top of the stem, leaving at least 5 inches of the stem end uncovered. Pack soil tightly and water the mound well. Keep the plant well watered for several weeks. Then check for the appearance of roots. When they are well established, make a quick clean cut through the stem, using a trowel or shovel to separate the layered herb from the original plant. Repot the new plant—take care not to disturb the roots. Keep the potted herb in a bright area away from direct sunlight. In a couple of months, you should notice leaves developing. Once they are well established, transplant the new plant.

Division: Most perennial herbs may be divided successfully, except those with deep tap roots. The best time to divide plants is early to midspring when growth starts or in early fall, about six weeks before the first full frost. Carefully dig up the plant. Try not to damage the root system. Keep as much dirt on the root ball as possible. Gently pull apart the roots to create two plants. If the roots are too strong to pull apart by hand, use a trowel or knife to divide them. Replant divided plants before they dry out. If you divide herbs in the fall, cut the tops back by about one half when dividing. Treat new plants as you would seedlings. Water them immediately, then daily for about a week. If tops wilt, cover with a plastic pot or move the plants to a shady location.

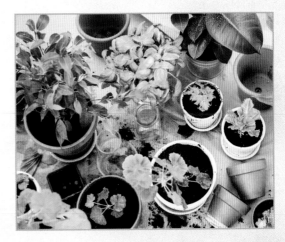

Purchase plants close to the time you want to set them in their beds or containers. If this is not possible, you may need to water the plants every day to keep them from drying out. Look for healthy plants that show no sign of insects or disease, are not too tall or spindly, and show signs of new growth. When you purchase herbs for cooking, smell the leaves. Water them as soon as they are home and keep them out of the sun until they revive.

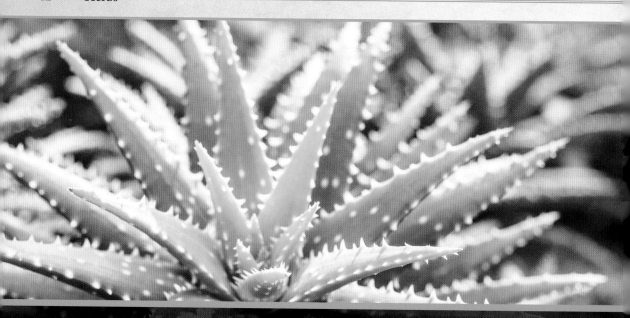

Aloe

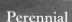

Perennial

Botanical Name: *Aloe vera* or *A. barbadensis*

Family: Liliaceae

Height: 1–5 ft. with flowering stalk

Spread: 1–3 ft.

Description: *Aloe vera* is the most common of the more than 300 species of aloe. Resistant to salt and drought, this very hardy herb can be found on rocky shorelines or dunes or intermingled with other vegetation just about anywhere. A common houseplant, aloe is characterized by pointed, fleshy leaves that exude a mucilaginous (gelatin-like) sap when broken. Aloe produces yellow to orange-red tubular flowers that grow to 1 inch. The herb is native to East Africa and widely cultivated in Egypt, the Near East, Bermuda, Spain, the Bahamas, the Caribbean, South America, southern Florida, and Texas.

Ease of care: Easy

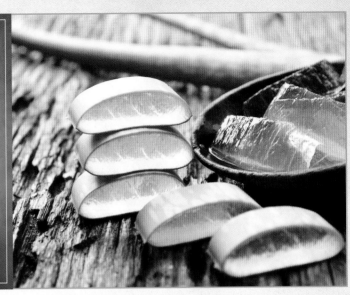

Break off a leaf, slice it down the middle, and rub the gel on the skin. To make a poultice of aloe, place the cut leaf on the burned or affected area, and wrap it with gauze. You can also apply store-bought gel or juice. Remove the yellow section if you juice your own aloe for internal use. Take up to 1/4 cup a day of pure aloe sweetened with fruit juice, or follow the directions for aloe juice.

Cultivation: Aloe needs neutral, average, well-drained soil with filtered sun to shade. In good soil and a warm climate, an aloe plant will thrive for years. It is not frost-hardy; it survives to zone 3. The plant's fleshy, spiky leaves make aloe a good ornamental garden plant.

Propagation: Aloe's tiny black seeds can germinate in about four weeks but often take many months. The best way to obtain new plants is to remove suckers or offshoots from the mother plant when they have grown 1 to 2 inches for an indoor plant and 6 to 8 inches for an outdoor plant. The herb takes two to three years to flower. Aloe is sold in nurseries throughout the country.

Uses: This common plant has many uncommon virtues. Cleopatra is said to have massaged fresh aloe gel into her skin every day to preserve her beauty. And, indeed, modern clinical studies show that aloe is one of the best herbs for soothing skin and healing burns, rashes, frostbite, and severe wounds. It is also used to treat eczema, dandruff, acne, ringworm, gum disease, and poison oak and ivy. Aloe is found commercially in a number of creams and lotions for softening and moisturizing skin. It works by inhibiting formation of tissue-injuring compounds that gather at the site of a skin injury. The plant contains chrysophanic acid, which is highly effective in healing abrasions. Some compounds from aloe show promise in the laboratory as potential cancer fighters.

Part used: Sap from fleshy leaves. Cut the outermost (oldest) leaves first. Aloe produces new leaves from its center.

Preservation: Use fresh leaves. To preserve, add vitamin C powder or liquid.

Precautions: Aloin, the yellow portion of aloe just under the leaf's peel, is a strong laxative that may cause severe cramping and diarrhea, so use aloe cautiously internally and always with a carminative such as ginger, fennel, or coriander. Commercial aloe juice has this property removed, so it is safe to drink as recommended on the bottle. People with diabetes should be careful using aloe—studies have shown it can reduce blood sugar levels.

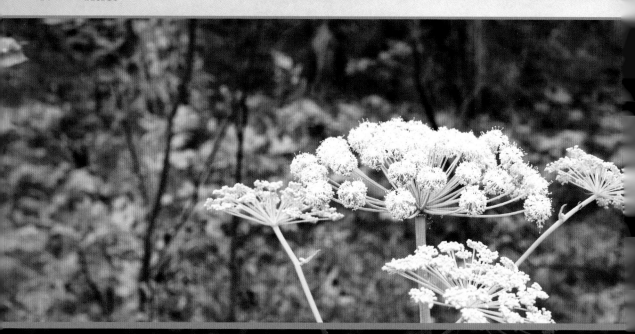

Angelica

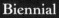

Biennial

Botanical Name: *Angelica archangelica*

Family: Apiaceae (Umbelliferae)

Height: 5–6 ft., in flower

Spread: 3 ft.

Description: This large, boldly attractive plant produces lush growth, making it a striking focal point for your garden. Angelica looks much like a very large celery or parsnip plant. This herb produces large white umbel flower heads and decorative yellow-green seedpods. Often you'll find angelica growing near seas, streams, and mountain brooks and in marshes, swamps, and moist meadows. It is native to Syria and possibly Europe but now cultivated elsewhere, including the United States.

Ease of care: Moderate

Cultivation: Angelica likes a cool, moist location and average to well-drained soil. It will grow in sun but prefers partial shade.

Propagation: Seeds must be no more than 6 months old to germinate. Sow them in late fall. Scatter seeds on top of soil and lightly cover with additional soil. Plant seeds directly in the garden, or transplant seedlings. Mature angelica plants do not like to be moved.

Uses: For centuries, people gathered angelica to ward off evil spirits. Early physicians prescribed angelica for a number of illnesses. Angelica syrup was taken as a digestive aid, and American Indians used angelica to treat lung congestion. Today angelica is used primarily to treat digestive and bronchial conditions and as an expectorant and cough suppressant. It has antibacterial, antifungal, and diaphoretic (induces sweating) properties. It also increases menstrual flow. In China, the Asian species is prescribed to improve liver function in people with cirrhosis and chronic hepatitis, to regulate menstruation, and to relieve menopausal symptoms. Studies have shown that compounds from Chinese angelica may also have cancer-fighting properties.

Commercially, angelica roots and seeds are used to flavor Benedictine and Chartreuse liqueurs, gin, vermouth, and some brands of tobacco. The herb's distinctive flavor is also found in fresh or dried leaves and stems. Add very small amounts of fresh leaves to salads, fruits, soups, stews, desserts, and pastries.

Part used: Leaves, seeds, stems, root

Preservation: Harvest roots during the plant's first fall or second spring, leaves throughout summer, stems anytime, and seeds when ripe. Stems may be candied or frozen. Hang-dry or freeze leaves.

Precautions: Don't attempt to gather wild species of angelica; they look a lot like water hemlock, which is extremely toxic. Angelica increases menstrual flow, so avoid it if you're pregnant. It contains chemicals called psoralens, which can cause some sensitive people to develop a rash when exposed to sunlight; some people get dermatitis when handling the leaves. Use small amounts of the herb since it can act strongly on the nervous system. If angelica causes you any problems, discontinue use.

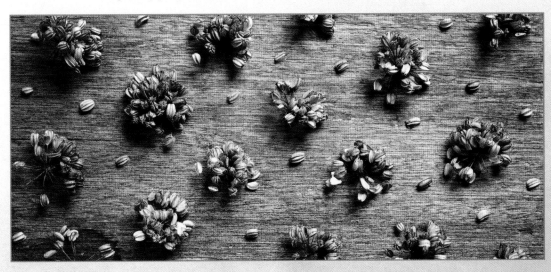

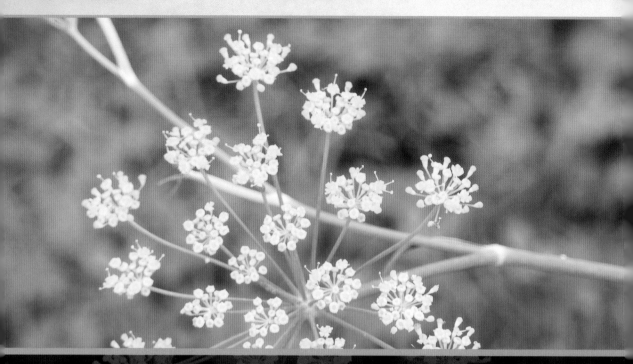

Anise

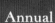

Annual

Botanical Name: *Pimpinella anisum*

Family: Apiaceae (Umbelliferae)

Height: 1–2 ft.

Spread: 8 in.

Description: Anise produces feathery leaves and a lacy flower umbel on slender, weak stems. The plant strongly resembles dill. It is native to Egypt and the Mediterranean region and widely cultivated in Europe, India, Mexico, Russia, and the United States.

Ease of care: Moderate

Cultivation: Anise prefers full sun and average, light, dry soil. Sow seed in the garden, or transplant seedlings when small. Like dill, anise grows best in rows or clumps so its weak multiple stems can support one another. It takes at least four months of warm, frost-free weather to grow seeds to maturity. In northern areas, the growing season is usually not long enough for anise to produce seeds.

Propagation: Sow seed in early spring. Because the plant produces a long taproot, it is difficult to transplant.

Uses: Anise has been considered a valuable herb since at least the 6th century BC. The Romans cultivated the plant for its distinctive fragrance and flavor, which is similar to licorice. They also used anise extensively as a medicine. For centuries, anise was used to induce a mother's milk to flow, to ease childbirth, and as an aphrodisiac. Today herbalists recommend anise to aid digestion and prevent gas. Because it loosens bronchial secretions and reduces coughing, anise is often found in cough syrups and lozenges. And the herb has some antimicrobial properties.

Anise is a prime ingredient in many ethnic cuisines, including Scandinavian, Greek, East Indian, Arabic, and Hispanic foods. The herb intensifies the flavor of pastries, cakes, and cookies, and it complements eggs, stewed fruit, cheese, spinach, and carrots. Use leaves whole in salads or as a garnish. Dried leaves make a pleasant-tasting tea, and the herb has been used to flavor liqueurs, including the well-known Greek ouzo. With its licorice-like taste, it is used to flavor most of the "licorice" candy in the United States and other candies as well.

Anise is rarely used alone but makes a great flavoring in teas and tinctures, and it is a popular addition to cough syrups.

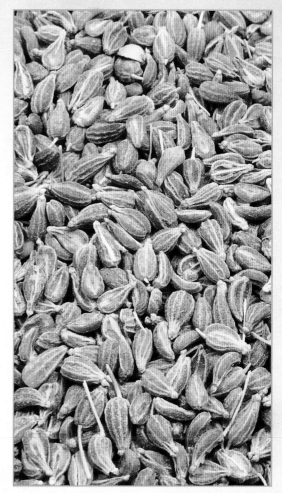

Part used: Seeds, leaves

Preservation: Harvest during late summer when seeds ripen. To collect seeds, hang-dry seed heads in paper bags in a warm, dry place. Store in tightly sealed containers.

Although anise has been recommended to treat morning sickness, the herb has an estrogen-like property. Pregnant women should avoid any herbs or drugs that might have an estrogenic effect. The essential oil can be narcotic and toxic, so use it carefully.

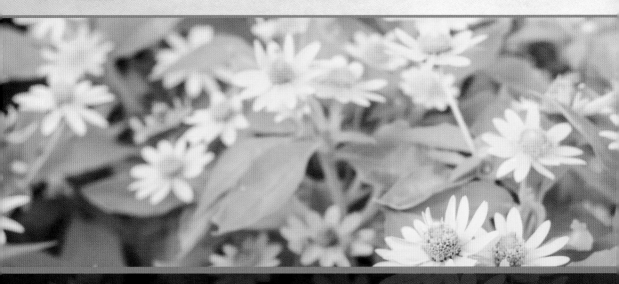

Arnica

Perennial

Botanical Name: *Arnica montana*

Family: Asteraceae (Compositae)

Height: 1–2 ft.

Spread: 10 in.

Description: Arnica, also called leopardsbane, mountain tobacco, and wolfsbane, is found in mountainous regions. The herb is indigenous to Europe and Siberia, but it has been naturalized in southwestern Canada and the western United States. Other species of arnica can be found from Alaska to New Mexico. The plant grows from a horizontal, dark brown root and produces round and hairy stems. These send up as many as three flower stalks with blossoms that resemble daisies and appear from June to August. Lance-shaped, bright green, and toothed, arnica's leaves appear somewhat hairy on their upper surfaces. The oval lower leaves grow to 5 inches long.

Ease of care: Moderate

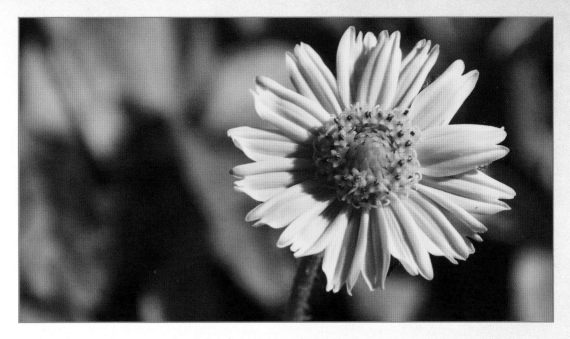

Cultivation: Arnica requires sandy, dry soil with humus and full sun. It prefers acidic soil but will grow in most beds as long as they are well drained. Some species of arnica tolerate light shade, including *A. cordifolia* and *A. latifolia*.

Propagation: New arnica plants may be produced by means of division, cuttings, or seeds.

Uses: The next time your calves ache after a strenuous run, try massaging them with an arnica liniment. European herbalists and American Indians have long recognized arnica's abilities to soothe and relax sore, stiff muscles. More than 100 commercial preparations in Germany contain arnica. It is also used to make homeopathic remedies. The flower is the most potent part of the plant, but sometimes the leaves are also used.

Arnica's healing powers have been attributed to two chemicals, helenalin and arnicin, which have anti-inflammatory, antiseptic, and pain-relieving properties. Arnica also increases blood circulation.

Part used: Flowers, leaves

Preservation: The plant is best used fresh. Gather flowers in midsummer, just as they reach their blooming peak. Preserve them in alcohol to make a liniment.

Precautions: The helenalin in arnica causes dermatitis in a few people after repeated applications. Discontinue use if you develop any skin problems. Otherwise, arnica is safe for topical use. But do not ingest arnica. Taken internally, the herb can irritate the kidneys and the digestive tract, cause dizziness, and elevate blood pressure. Arnica is available in tinctures, salves, and ointments to treat minor wounds, sprains, and bruises. You can lay a compress made with arnica tea or the diluted tincture on such injuries, or place a compress on the stomach to relieve abdominal pain. To make an arnica oil, heat 1 ounce of flowers in 10 ounces of any vegetable oil for several hours on low heat. Strain and let the oil cool before applying it to bruises or sore muscles.

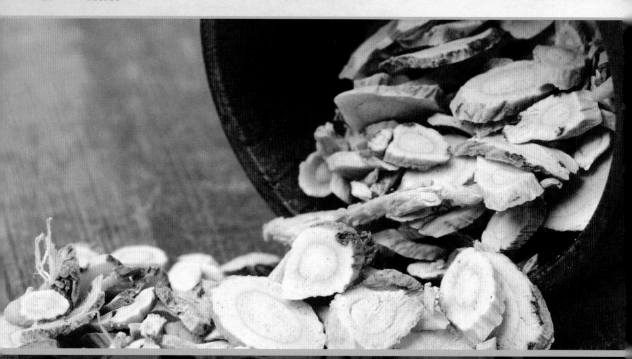

Astragalus

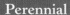

Perennial

Botanical Name: *Astragalus membranaceus*

Family: Fabaceae (Leguminosae)

Height: 4 ft.

Spread: 1 1/2 ft.

Description: Known as milk-vetch in the West and *huang qi* in the East, this plant produces symmetrical oblong, pointed leaves. Astragalus is a member of the legume family, which includes lentils, beans, clover, and licorice.

Ease of care: Moderate

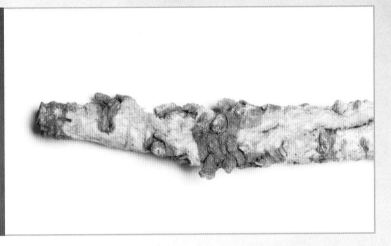

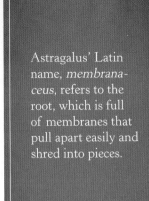

Astragalus' Latin name, *membranaceus*, refers to the root, which is full of membranes that pull apart easily and shred into pieces.

Cultivation: Astragalus is not yet found in most herb gardens, but it is gaining popularity as its use in North America increases. In Asia, it is cultivated commercially or gathered in the wild.

Propagation: Astragalus roots may be divided or grown from seed.

Uses: Here in the West we're just beginning to appreciate the healing properties of astragalus, an herb that has been revered in Asia for more than 2,000 years. Compiled by Chinese physicians in the first century AD, *The Divine Husbandman's Classic of the Materia Medica* lists astragalus as its number-one health-giving plant. Chinese physicians believe that astragalus is a tonic for the lung and spleen. Because of its immune-system-enhancing properties, astragalus is often prescribed for people with "wasting" diseases such as fatigue or loss of appetite due to chronic illness, or for people who need to strengthen their body's systems. It is also used to treat chronic diarrhea. It is not uncommon in China to use astragalus extracts to fight several kinds of cancer. It is used in Chinese hospitals to lessen the side effects of chemotherapy and radiation; studies have also found it improves survival rates of cancer patients.

Astragalus is an excellent diuretic. It lowers fevers and has a beneficial effect on the digestive system. Other illnesses for which herbalists use astragalus include arthritis; diabetes; inflammation in the urinary tract; prolapsed uterus, stomach, or anus; uterine bleeding and weakness; water retention; and skin wounds that refuse to heal.

Astragalus' ability to lower blood pressure is probably due to the gamma-aminobutyric acid it contains, which dilates blood vessels. Other chemicals in the root have been found to strengthen the lungs.

In commercial preparations, astragalus is often combined with other herbs. That's because astragalus appears to act as a synergist—it enhances or strengthens the effects of companion ingredients. Chinese herbalists combine it with Chinese red sage, licorice, ligustrum, codonopsis, schisandra, and atractylodes. In the West, astragalus is often combined with echinacea, ginseng, licorice, and garlic.

Part used: Root

Preservation: The root is harvested in the fall and dried.

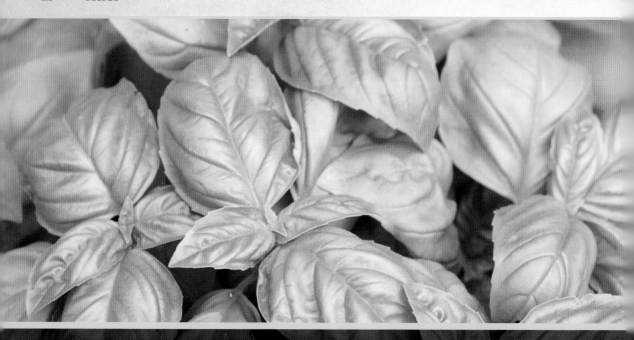

Basil

Annual

Botanical Name: *Ocimum basilicum*

Family: Lamiaceae (Labiatae)

Height: 1 1/2 ft.

Spread: 10 in.

Description: Basil produces a neat, dense growth, with bright-green, triangular leaves. You can even clip basil into a neat hedge. Basil is native to India, Africa, and Asia and cultivated in France, Egypt, Hungary, Indonesia, Morocco, Greece, Bulgaria, the former Yugoslavian nations, and Italy. In the United States, it is widely grown in California and in kitchen gardens all over the country.

Ease of care: Easy

Cultivation: Basil prefers full sun and semi-rich, moist soil. It will grow in partial shade but gets "leggy" (it grows sparsely and doesn't fill out).

Propagation: Sow seeds when soil is warm, or get a head start by planting seeds indoors and transplanting seedlings after the danger of frost is past.

Uses: A member of the mint family, basil is recommended to aid digestion and expel gas. It's also good for treating stomach cramps, vomiting, and constipation. It has been found to be more effective than drugs to relieve nausea from chemotherapy and radiation. In India, *O. sanctum* is used to prevent stomach ulcers, colitis, asthma, and high blood pressure. Basil has a slight sedative action and sometimes is recommended for nervous headaches and anxiety. Studies show that extracts of basil seeds have antibacterial properties. Basil contains vitamins A and C as well as antioxidants, which prevent cell damage. One study found that basil increases production of disease-fighting antibodies up to 20 percent. It also combats the herpesvirus.

In Malaysia, basil is used to expel intestinal worms. Clinical studies show that basil essential oil is, indeed, effective in killing parasites.

In the kitchen, basil's rich, spicy flavor—something like pepper with a hint of mint and cloves—works wonders in pesto, tomato sauce, salads, cheese dishes, eggs, stews, vinegars, and all sorts of vegetables. Often you'll find basil in ethnic cuisines, particularly those of Italy and Thailand.

Strongly fragrant, basil is used in sachets and potpourri. A basil infusion used as a hair rinse adds luster to the hair and helps treat acne and itching skin. Basil essential oil is found in perfumes and toilet waters, lotions, shampoos, and soaps. Added to the bath, it produces an invigorating soak.

Part used: Leaves

Preservation: Take prunings and use fresh leaves any time. Harvest basil when buds are about to blossom—when the plant is at its flavor peak—and hang-dry. Basil retains its flavor best when frozen or stored in oil or vinegar.

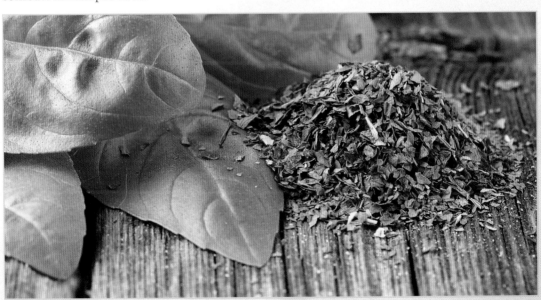

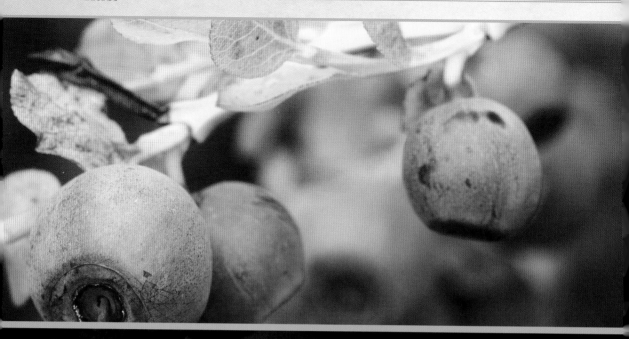

Bilberry

Perennial

Botanical Name: *Vaccinium myrtillus*

Family: Ericaceae

Height: 1–2 ft.

Spread: 3–4 ft.

Description: Bilberry is a deciduous shrub with thin, creeping stems. Leaves are bright green, alternate, and oval. Flowers are pale green to pink and appear from late spring to late summer, followed by purple fruit. Native to Europe, northern Asia, and North America, the herb is found in woodlands, forests, and moorlands. One of more than 100 members of the genus *Vaccinium*, bilberry is related to blueberries and huckleberries.

Ease of care: Moderate

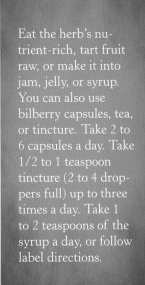

Eat the herb's nutrient-rich, tart fruit raw, or make it into jam, jelly, or syrup. You can also use bilberry capsules, tea, or tincture. Take 2 to 6 capsules a day. Take 1/2 to 1 teaspoon tincture (2 to 4 droppers full) up to three times a day. Take 1 to 2 teaspoons of the syrup a day, or follow label directions.

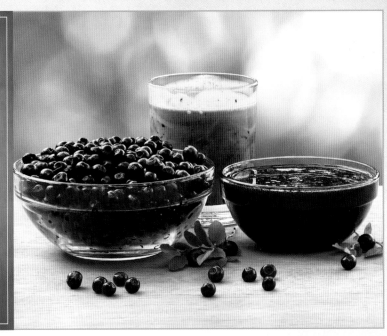

Cultivation: A wild herb, bilberry requires acidic, peaty soil and sun or filtered shade.

Propagation: New plants may be grown from rooted cuttings in spring or fall.

Uses: Bilberry contains vitamins A and C and was a folk remedy in Scandinavia to prevent scurvy and treat nausea and indigestion. The berries were once steeped in gin and taken as a digestive tonic. They are a popular Russian remedy for colitis and stomach ulcers because they decrease inflammation in the intestines and protect the lining of the digestive tract. The herb has astringent, antiseptic, and tonic properties, making it useful as a treatment for diarrhea.

Berries contain flavonoid anthocyanidins, which have a potent antioxidant action and protect body tissues, particularly blood vessels. Several studies have shown that bilberry extracts stimulate blood vessels to release a substance that helps dilate (open) veins and arteries. Bilberries may keep platelets from clumping, thus preventing clotting and improving circulation. The berry may help prevent many diabetes-related conditions caused by poor circulation.

Because they contain a substance that slightly lowers blood sugar, the leaves are a folk remedy to manage diabetes. However, you should not use the leaves to self-treat diabetes. German researchers have investigated the leaves as a treatment for gout and rheumatism.

Bilberry preparations may be particularly useful for treating eye conditions and have been prescribed for diabetic retinopathy, cataracts, night blindness, and macular degeneration. In England, World War II pilots were given bilberry jam to improve their eyesight. Modern European prescription medications that contain bilberry are used to improve eyesight and circulation.

Part used: Fruit, leaves

Preservation: Gather fruit when ripe and use fresh, or freeze.

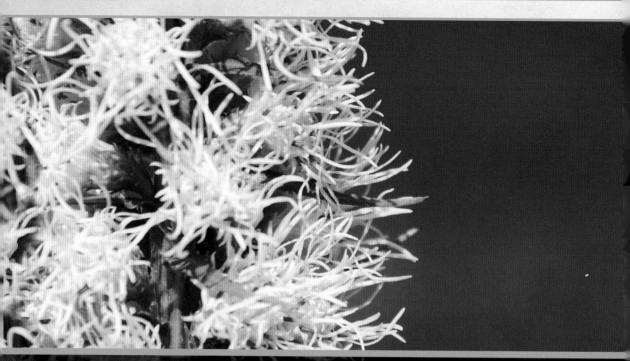

Black Cohosh

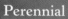

Perennial

Botanical Name: *Cimicifuga racemosa*

Family: Ranunculaceae

Height: 3–6 ft. (flower stalk)

Spread: 2 ft.

Description: Related to buttercup, larkspur, and peony, black cohosh is a leafy herb with knotty black roots and a smooth stem. Also known as snakeroot, the plant produces small, multiple white flowers in midsummer on tall stalks. Black cohosh grows in the eastern United States and Canada.

Ease of care: Moderate

Cultivation: Black cohosh is a wild plant that prefers rich soil and forest conditions. Seeds take two to four weeks to germinate and are best stratified.

Propagation: Sow seed in spring; divide roots in spring or fall.

Uses: North American Indians used black cohosh to treat fatigue, sore throat, arthritis, and rattlesnake bite, but the herb's primary use historically was as a medicine to ease childbirth. Nineteenth-century American herbalists also recommended black cohosh for fever and menstrual cramps. Black cohosh is a diuretic, expectorant, astringent, and sedative, but today it is most often recommended for treating symptoms of menopause. The herb seems to have an estrogenic effect by binding to estrogen receptors in the body. Black cohosh contains salicylic acid (the main ingredient of aspirin) and has been used for a variety of muscular, pelvic, and rheumatic pains, especially those caused by nervous tension. Herbalists in China use a related species, *C. foetida*, to treat headache, measles, and gynecologic problems.

Part used: Root

Preservation: Harvest the roots in the fall; cut them lengthwise and dry.

Precautions: An overdose of black cohosh may cause dizziness, diarrhea, abdominal pain, vomiting, visual dimness, headache, tremors, and a depressed heart rate. Don't use it if you have a heart condition. Because the herb seems to affect hormones, don't use it if you're pregnant.

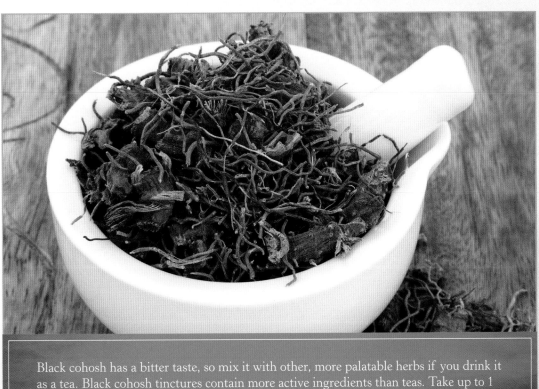

Black cohosh has a bitter taste, so mix it with other, more palatable herbs if you drink it as a tea. Black cohosh tinctures contain more active ingredients than teas. Take up to 1 teaspoon (4 droppers full) of tincture or 2 cups of tea a day.

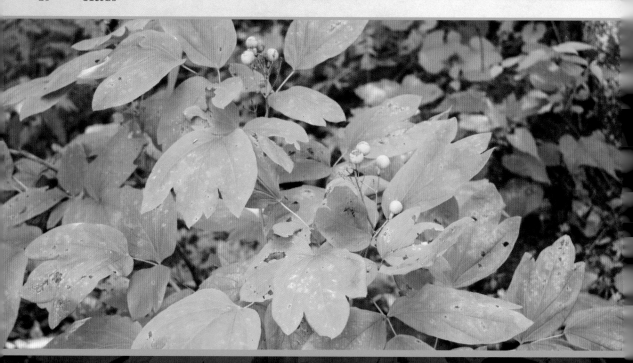

Blue Cohosh

Perennial

Botanical Name: *Caulophyllum thalictroides*

Family: Berberidaceae

Height: 1–3 ft.

Spread: 1 1/2 ft.

Description: Blue cohosh is a bluish-green, deciduous plant that flowers in June to August, producing yellow-green clusters of blooms on tall stalks. Blue cohosh is native to North America and grows from New Brunswick to Manitoba and south to Alabama. You may encounter blue cohosh in woods and along stream banks.

Ease of care: Moderate

Cultivation: The herb likes rich, moist, humusy soil and shade.

Propagation: Sow seeds in spring; if you plant them in fall, they may germinate the following spring. Divide rhizomes in spring or fall. Seeds and rhizomes are available through mail order from wild flower and herb sources.

Uses: American Indians considered blue cohosh a panacea for women's ailments. Over the centuries and up to the present time, the herb has been used to treat uterine abnormalities and relieve menstrual cramps. Before the introduction of forceps, American obstetricians used blue cohosh to help induce labor.

In the past, blue cohosh was used to treat bronchitis, rheumatism, and irregular menstruation. It was also combined with other herbs, including motherwort and partridge berry, for women in the last few weeks of pregnancy to promote smooth labor.

Part used: Rhizome

Preservation: Make the dried rhizome into tinctures, decoctions, or capsules.

Precautions: Blue cohosh contains several strong compounds. It can constrict coronary blood vessels, so do not use it if you have a history of stroke or have high blood pressure, heart disease, or diabetes. The powdered rhizome irritates mucous membranes, so handle it with care; don't inhale it or get it in your eyes. And don't take blue cohosh during labor unless you are working with an herbalist or midwife knowledgeable about herbs. Above all, do not eat the berries: They are poisonous!

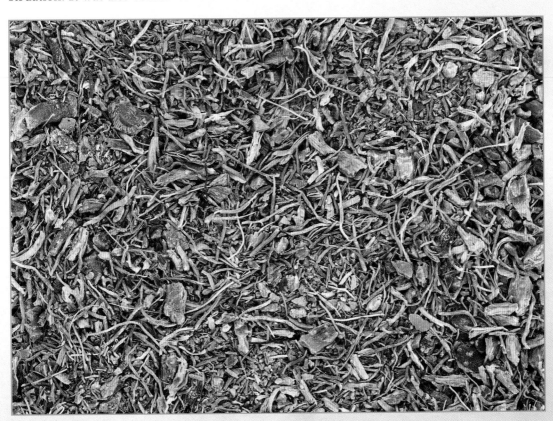

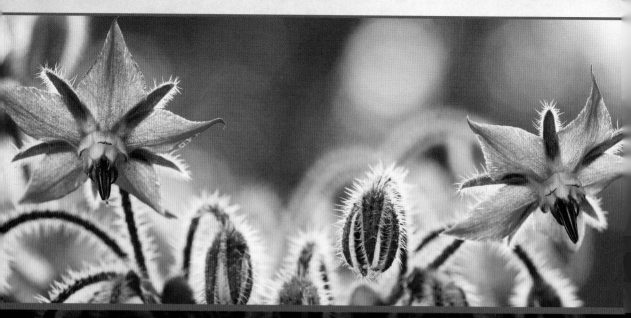

Borage

Annual (with Biennial characteristics)

Botanical Name: *Borago officinalis*

Family: Boraginaceae

Height: 2–2 1/2 ft.

Spread: 1 1/2 ft.

Description: The herb's basal rosette of long, spear-shaped leaves produces tall stems covered with attractive, bright-blue, star-shaped flowers that hang downward. All parts of the plant are covered with bristly "hairs." Borage is a nice addition to any flower garden. Although usually grown as an annual, the plant will often overwinter in mild climates for a second growing season. Borage is native to Europe, Asia Minor, northern Europe, and Africa. It has become naturalized in Great Britain and is found widely in North America, often in waste places and along roads.

Ease of care: Easy

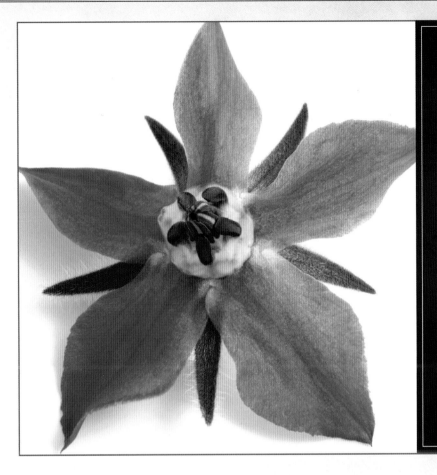

Borage is safe to use in small amounts, but you should limit your intake; the herb contains the same type of alkaloids as comfrey. Some researchers strongly suggest not eating the leaves, which contain higher amounts of pyrrolizidine alkaloids than the flowers do. Use the flowers in foods and the leaves in poultices.

Cultivation: Borage prefers a dry, sunny location in poor to ordinary, well-drained soil. It is difficult to transplant; if you must do so, move the plant when it is young.

Propagation: Sow seed in early spring or late fall.

Uses: Celtic warriors drank borage wine because they believed it gave them courage. Romans thought borage produced a sense of elation and well-being. The Greeks turned to the herb when their spirits sagged. Today, herbalists consider borage a diuretic, demulcent, and emollient, and prescribe the plant to treat depression, fevers, bronchitis, and diarrhea. The malic acid and potassium nitrate it contains may be responsible for its diuretic effects. Poultices of leaves may be useful in cooling and soothing skin and reducing inflammation and swelling. The plant also has expectorant properties.

The crisp flavor of borage flowers complements cheese, fish, poultry, most vegetables, salads, iced beverages, pickles, and salad dressings. You can eat small amounts of young leaves: Steam well as you would spinach so the leaves are no longer prickly. You can also candy the flowers.

Part used: Flowers, leaves

Preservation: Pick blossoms as they open and use them fresh or candied. Young leaves are good for fresh use. Because borage flowers lose much of their flavor when dried, preserve them in vinegar to use later.

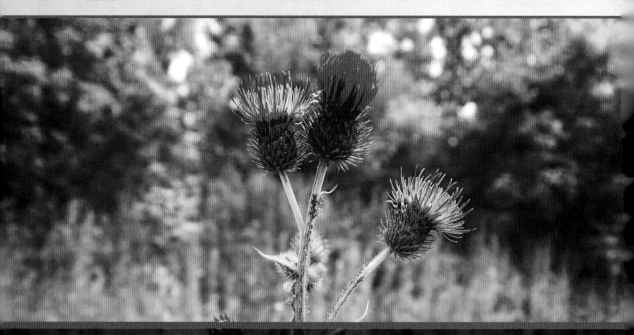

Burdock

Biennial (may be grown as an Annual)

Botanical Name: *Arctium lappa, A. minus*

Family: Asteraceae (Compositae)

Height: To 6 ft.

Spread: 3 ft.

Description: This stout, coarse herb has many branches, each topped by numerous flowers, which appear in summer. The seed burrs cling to anything that rubs against them. The large leaves grow to 20 inches. Native to Eurasia, burdock has become naturalized throughout North America. You're likely to find burdock in fields and vacant lots, especially in damp areas.

Ease of care: Easy

Cultivation: A wild plant, burdock prefers average, moist, deep, loose, and well-drained soil and full sun, but it will grow in filtered sun.

Propagation: Burdock is grown easily from seed sown in the spring. Seedlings transplant well, but older plants are more difficult to relocate because they produce long taproots.

Uses: If you've ever returned from an outdoor romp with your pet and discovered burrs clinging tenaciously to the cuffs of your trousers and your pet's fur, you've encountered burdock, an herb whose primary use is as a blood purifier. The root is also considered a diuretic, diaphoretic, and laxative. It has also been used to treat psoriasis, acne, and other skin conditions. Research has found that several compounds in burdock root inhibit growth of bacteria and fungi. A poultice of leaves is effective in healing bruises, burns, and swellings. The Chinese also use burdock root to treat colds, flu, measles, and constipation and burdock seeds to treat skin problems. Herbalists use burdock to treat liver disorders.

Burdock also contains a substance called inulin, a starch that is easily digested. Burdock root tastes like a marriage of potato and celery; eat it fresh or steamed. Eat young stalks raw or steam them as you would asparagus. Burdock root is a staple of Japanese cuisine and sold in Japanese grocery stores, often under the name gobo root.

Part used: Root, leaves, seeds

Preservation: Dig roots in the plant's first fall or second spring; use them fresh or dry. Gather leaves before flowers bloom. Gather seeds after they ripen.

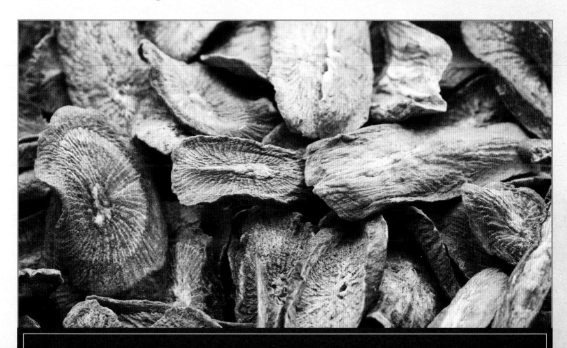

Burdock may be consumed as a vegetable, dried for tea, or tinctured. Drink up to 2 cups of tea a day. Take 1/2 to 1 teaspoon tincture up to three times a day.

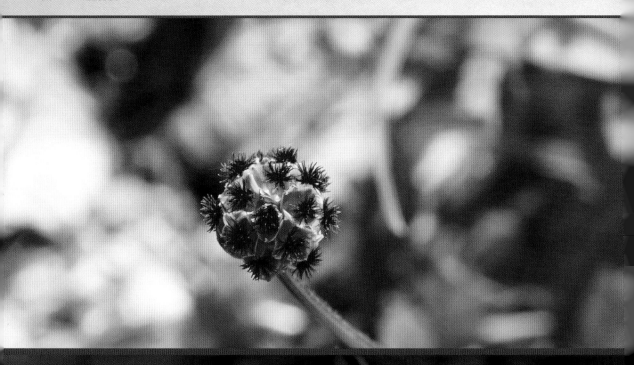

Burnet

Perennial

Botanical Name: *Poterium sanguisorba*

Family: Rosaceae

Height: 1 1/2 ft., in flower

Spread: 1 ft.

Description: A ground-hugging rosette of dark green leaves forms the plant, from which thin, 1 to 1 1/2-foot stems arise to produce handsome purple flower heads. Burnet makes a good edging plant. Also called salad burnet, the plant is native to western Asia and Europe and has become naturalized in North America.

Ease of care: Easy

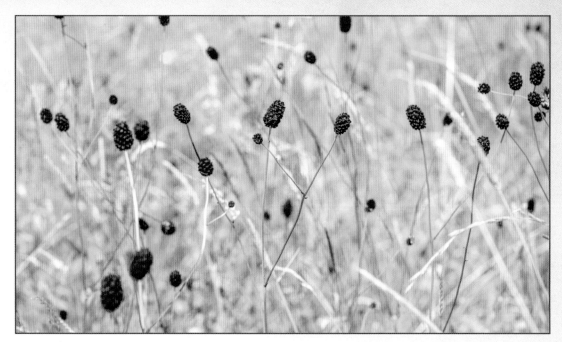

Cultivation: Burnet prefers full sun in average soil, although rich soil improves its flavor, making it less bitter. Burnet prefers an alkaline soil; if your soil is very acidic, add lime.

Propagation: Sow seed. Burnet self-sows easily after its first planting.

Uses: Herbalists have used burnet for at least 2,000 years. Useful to control bleeding, burnet's name, in fact, means "to drink up blood." Nineteenth-century Shakers used burnet for healing wounds. And the herb is considered helpful in treating vaginal discharges and diarrhea. Burnet leaves contain vitamin C and tannins; the latter gives it astringent properties. It relieves indigestion and diarrhea. Practitioners of traditional Chinese medicine use the root topically on wounds and burns to reduce inflammation and the risk of infection. It is also used to treat gum disease. While burnet is rarely used medicinally in North America, Europeans and Russians still use it in their folk medicine. It is used to heal ulcerative colitis as a folk remedy in Northern Europe and Russia. Apparently, its medicinal properties are due to more than simply the astringent tannins it contains. Russian research shows that the leaves improve circulation to the uterus, especially in pregnant women. The leaves also have immune-enhancing properties that may help correct some abnormalities during pregnancy.

In the kitchen, use tender, young, well-chopped leaves in salads, vinegars, butters, and iced beverages. Add leaves to vinegars, marinades, and cheese spreads. And flowers make attractive garnishes.

Part used: Leaves, flowers

Preservation: Burnet does not dry well. Harvest leaves in early autumn and preserve them in vinegar.

Precautions: Although Russian studies show its value during pregnancy, use only small amounts unless a health practitioner recommends it.

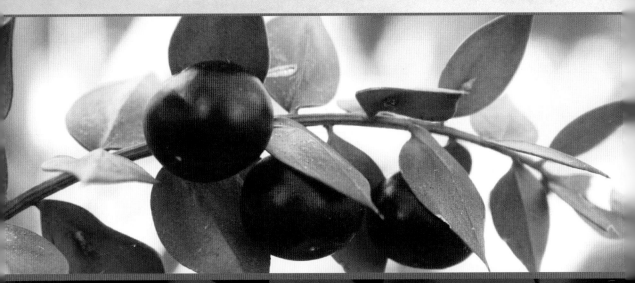

Butcher's Broom

Perennial

Botanical Name: *Ruscus aculeatus*

Family: Liliaceae

Height: 4 ft.

Spread: To 3 ft.

Description: For 300 years—from the 16th to 19th centuries—butcher's broom was associated with the meat industry. Butchers used the leaves to repel vermin and animals. Later, they made "brooms" from the plant to scrub chopping blocks. With its waxy green leaves and scarlet berries, butcher's broom has been used to decorate meats at Christmas; indeed, another name for the herb is box holly. Found naturally from the Azores to Iran, butcher's broom is an erect evergreen, with prickly leaves and whitish or pinkish flowers that appear from midautumn to late spring. Its round berries are scarlet or yellow. Butcher's broom is found in woodland thickets on poor, dry, rocky soil.

Ease of care: Easy

Cultivation: Cultivate butcher's broom in regular garden soil. An attractive plant, it is available at many nurseries, sold as an ornamental.

Propagation: Seeds, cuttings

Uses: Butcher's broom enjoys a venerable history as a medicinal herb. The ancient Greeks recommended butcher's broom for treating kidney stones, gout, and jaundice.

Butcher's broom has experienced a comeback in recent years. There is some evidence it may have value in treating circulatory problems, such as varicose veins and hemorrhoids. In German studies, it decreased the inflammation of varicose veins, helped to tighten them, and encouraged the blood to flow up the legs. In addition to strengthening blood vessels, the plant reduces fever and increases urine flow.

Drink 2 to 3 cups of tea a day to treat circulation problems or take 1/2 teaspoon tincture (2 droppers full) a day. Butcher's broom is often combined with other herbs that are good for circulation, such as gingko and hawthorn.

Part used: Leaves

Preservation: Harvest leaves when the plant goes into flower. Dry or use fresh.

Precautions: Butcher's broom may elevate blood pressure; do not use if you have high blood pressure.

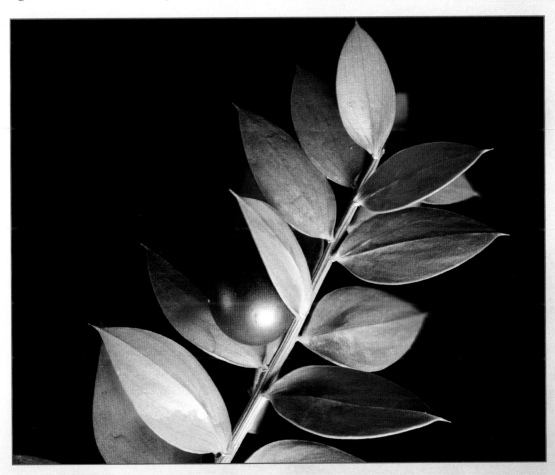

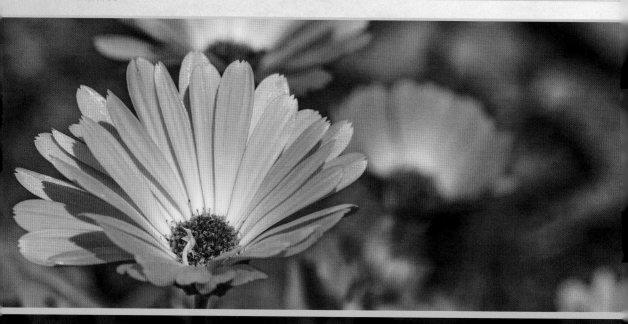

Calendula

Annual

Botanical Name: *Calendula officinalis*

Family: Asteraceae (Compositae)

Height: 1–2 ft.

Spread: 1 ft.

Description: Calendula produces coarse, bright green leaves attached to brittle stems. The plant grows rapidly and blooms abundantly throughout summer, until the first frost. Also called pot marigold, the herb's flower colors range from bright yellow to vivid orange. (It is not a true marigold.) Calendula is a cheerful addition to any garden and makes an attractive potted plant. Calendula is found naturally from the Canary Islands through southern and central Europe. It is cultivated widely around the world.

Ease of care: Easy

Cultivation: Calendula enjoys full sun and average, well-drained soil. Be on the lookout for insects, which adore calendula.

Propagation: Sow seed outdoors in early spring or indoors about seven weeks before the last frost.

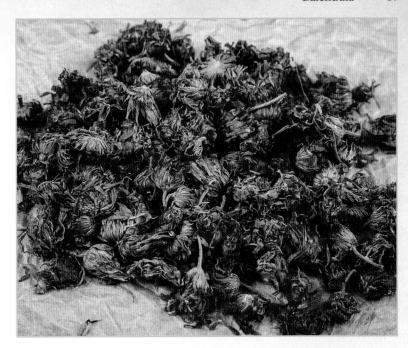

Uses: The Romans grew these plants to treat scorpion bites. In accordance with the Doctrine of Signatures, calendula's yellow flowers were believed to be an effective treatment for jaundice. The herb is used today to treat wounds, skin conditions, and peptic and duodenal ulcers. Calendula's primary use is to heal the skin and reduce swelling. Apply calendula to sores, cuts, bruises, burns, and rashes. It even soothes the discomfort of measles and chicken pox—simply make a double strength tea and wash over the skin eruptions. It also helps prevent and relieve diaper rash. Calendula induces sweating, increases urination, and aids digestion. Researchers have found that compounds in calendula may be useful in treating cancer. It has traditionally been used to treat tonsillitis and any condition related to swollen lymph glands, including breast cancer. It is also an excellent treatment for infection due to *Candida albicans*. Calendula tincture is used topically on varicose veins, bruises, and sprains.

In the kitchen, add a few calendula flowers to salads and sandwiches. Powdered yellow flowers may substitute for saffron's color (they once were used to color butter, custards, and liqueurs), although go easy—they have a bitter taste. The flowers produce a bright yellow dye and are commercially grown. Dry flowers for potpourri. A calendula rinse brings out highlights in hair. It is a popular ingredient in skin cream and lotions, baby oils, and salves.

To treat thrush, an infection with the Candida organism that appears in the mouth, swab the area with a tincture diluted in an equal amount of distilled water. Calendula is rarely drunk as a tea. A strong infusion, however, makes a good compress. For a poultice, mash fresh flowers and apply to the skin. To make calendula oil, crush dried or wilted flowers, then heat in olive oil for a few hours on low heat. Strain.

Part used: Flowers

Preservation: Dry whole flowers or remove petals from their green backs and spread them thinly on screens to dry. Stir while drying to prevent petals from molding.

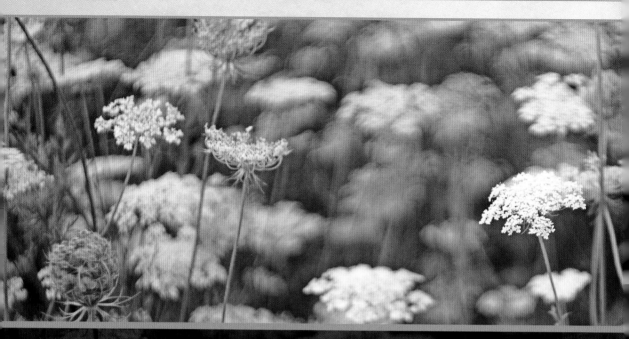

Caraway

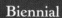

Biennial

Botanical Name: *Carum carvi*

Family: Apiaceae (Umbelliferae)

Height: 2 ft.

Spread: 8 in.

Description: Although caraway is a biennial, some varieties behave as annuals, going to seed in their first year. Caraway is characterized by fine-cut leaves that resemble the foliage of carrots. White umbels develop in the plant's second year to produce distinctively flavored seeds. Native to the Middle East, Asia, and central Europe, caraway has become naturalized in North America.

Ease of care: Moderate

Cultivation: Caraway grows best in a light, average, well-drained soil in full sun, although it tolerates partial shade. Plant in place; caraway produces a long taproot and does not transplant easily.

Propagation: Sow seeds outdoors in early spring or late summer.

Uses: Caraway seeds were found in ancient tombs, indicating the plant was used at least 5,000 years ago. As a medicine, caraway is used—most often as a cordial—to relieve an upset stomach and dispel gas. Caraway water has long been given to babies with colic. A compress soaked in a strong infusion or the powdered and moistened seed relieves swelling and bruising. But you may be most familiar with caraway from eating sauerkraut, rye crackers, and rye bread—foods that rely heavily on its strong aroma and taste. Add caraway seeds to beef dishes, stews, and breads. Add leaves to salads and soups. The herb complements eggs, cheese, sauces, barley, oats, pork, and fish, as well as cabbage, beets, spinach, potatoes, peas, cauliflower, turnips, and zucchini. Cooking it a long time can make it bitter, so add caraway no more than 30 minutes before a dish is done. It also makes children's medicines more tasty. The essential oil is added to soaps, cosmetics, perfumes, and mouthwashes and used to flavor liqueurs in Germany, Scandinavia, and Russia.

Part used: Leaves, seeds, root

Preservation: Cut plants at ground level when seeds ripen. Hang-dry seed heads in paper bags in a cool, dry place. Store seeds in tightly sealed containers. In its first fall or spring, dig up roots, clean, and store in a cool, dark area.

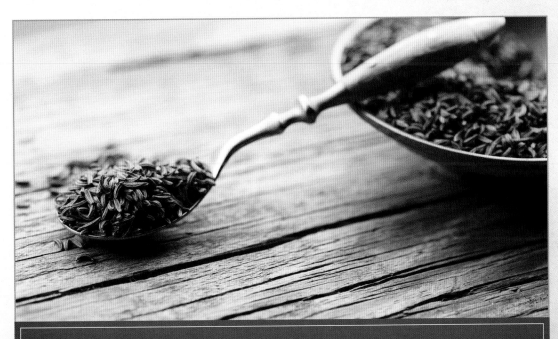

The most popular way to use caraway medicinally is in food. It is rare to find anyone using it by itself as a tincture or tea, but sometimes it flavors tinctures or syrups.

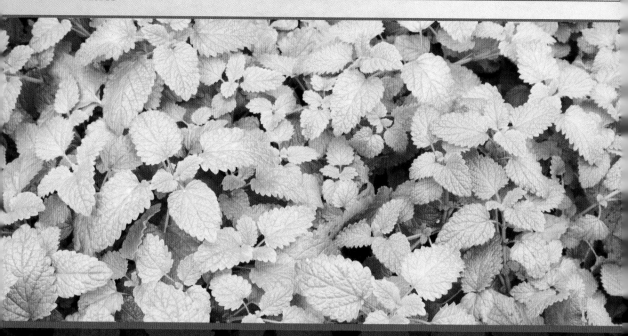

Catnip

Perennial

Botanical Name: *Nepeta cataria*

Family: Lamiaceae (Labiatae)

Height: 3–4 ft.

Spread: 2 ft.

Description: Also called catmint, this herb produces fuzzy, gray-green, triangular leaves in pairs along abundant branches. The leaves give off a pungent scent when crushed. From July through September, catnip produces white flowers with purple or pink spots. The herb is native to the Eurasian region and naturalized throughout North America and elsewhere.

Ease of care: Easy

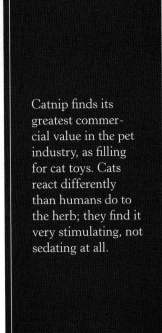

Catnip finds its greatest commercial value in the pet industry, as filling for cat toys. Cats react differently than humans do to the herb; they find it very stimulating, not sedating at all.

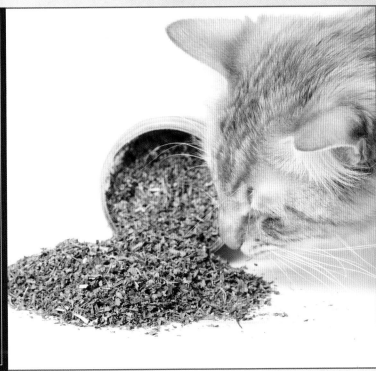

Cultivation: Catnip grows well in full sun to partial shade, in average to sandy, well-drained soil.

Propagation: Sow seed in spring or fall; take cuttings in early summer.

Uses: Your cat may go crazy over catnip, but the herb has actually been used as a mild sedative for about 2,000 years. The Romans harvested catnip, and colonists carried the herb to America, where it quickly became naturalized. Catnip tea aids digestion, promotes sleep, and treats colds, nervousness, and headaches. Its most important use is as a sedative that is safe enough even for children and the elderly. Catnip contains sedative constituents similar to valerian, another popular herbal relaxant. One of catnip's most famous uses is to treat colic in babies—a condition for which it has been used for hundreds of years. It also makes a good tea for treating indigestion associated with anxiety or nervousness. The tea treats measles and chicken pox when used both internally and topically. An infusion applied to the skin relieves hives and other rashes. The herb increases perspiration, reduces fevers, and increases menstrual flow. The herb's fragrance also repels some insects.

Catnip is usually combined with other herbs in a tea or tincture. For indigestion or for use as a gentle sedative, mix it with chamomile and lemon balm. For a stronger muscle and nerve relaxant, mix it with valerian or skullcap. Take up to 4 cups of tea or 1 teaspoon (4 droppers full) of tincture a day.

Part used: Leaves

Preservation: Gather leaves in late summer just before the plant blooms. Hang-dry plants, remove leaves from stems, and store in airtight containers.

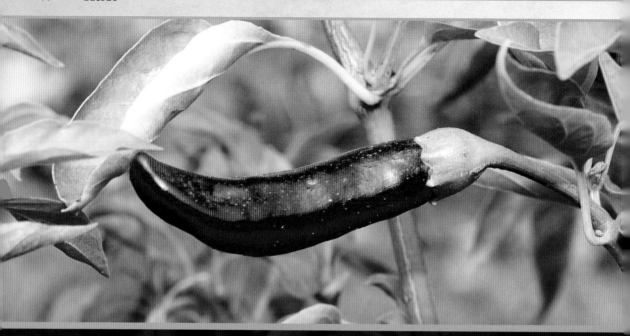

Cayenne Pepper

Perennial

Botanical Name: *Capsicum annuum*

Family: Solanaceae

Height: 1–3 ft.

Spread: 1 ft.

Description: Cayenne's angular branches and stems may look purplish. Its red fruits are extremely hot. Flowers, which appear in drooping clusters on long stems, are star-shaped and yellowish-white. Leaves are long and elliptical. Cayenne grows naturally in the tropics, but gardeners in most parts of the United States can grow it with success.

Ease of care: Easy

Cultivation: Unless you live in an area that rarely experiences freezing temperatures, it's best to plant cayenne in containers you can bring inside when temperatures drop, or grow it as an annual. The plant grows best in rich soil. If your soil is average, fertilize it with compost, rock phosphate, or wood ashes. Cayenne likes full sun. Give your plants lots of water during early stages of growth. Mulching protects them from drought.

Propagation: Because cayenne has a long growing season (up to 18 weeks), start plants indoors if propagating from seed. Transplant seedlings 12 to 18 inches apart, and allow 3 feet between rows.

Uses: Cayenne has many medicinal uses. The main ingredient in cayenne is capsaicin, a powerful stimulant responsible for the pepper's heat. Although it can set your mouth on fire, cayenne, ironically, is good for your digestive system and is now known to help heal ulcers. It reduces substance P, a chemical that carries pain messages from the skin's nerve endings, so it reduces pain when applied topically. A cayenne cream is now in use to treat psoriasis, postsurgical pain, shingles, and nerve damage from diabetes. It may even help you burn off extra pounds. Researchers in England have found that about 1/4 ounce of cayenne burns from 45 to 76 calories by increasing metabolism.

Taking cayenne internally stabilizes blood pressure. You can apply powdered, dry cayenne as a poultice over wounds to stop bleeding. And in the kitchen, cayenne spices up any food it touches.

Part used: Fruit

Preservation: Pick cayenne peppers after the fruits have turned red. Dry immediately and store in a cool, dry place. You can also freeze cayenne peppers or preserve them in oil or vinegar.

Precautions: Overexposure to the skin can produce pain, dizziness, and a rapid pulse. Alcohol or fat, such as whole milk, neutralizes the reaction. If you touch a pepper and then rub your eyes or nose, you could inflame those sensitive tissues.

Add a pinch of cayenne powder to other herbal infusions to treat colds and influenza. Simmer 3 tablespoons cayenne in 1 cup of cider vinegar. Do not strain. Shake before using. Take 1 teaspoon (4 droppers full) straight or add it to 1/2 cup warm water or tea for colds, flu, or sore throat. You can also combine cayenne with other heating herbs such as peppermint, eucalyptus, cinnamon, rosemary, and thyme in liniments for sore muscles or lung congestion.

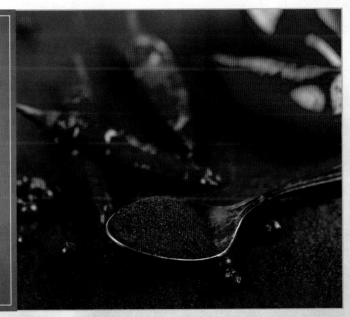

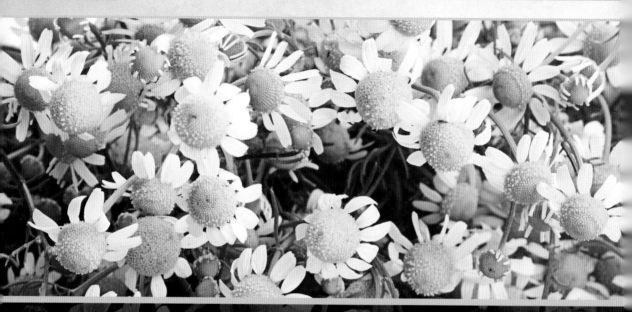

Chamomile, German

Annual

Botanical Name: *Matricaria recutita*

Family: Asteraceae (Compositae)

Height: 2 ft.

Spread: 4–6 in.

Description: These small, fine-leaved plants look almost like ferns, but the herb's abundant, small, daisy-type flowers have an apple scent. German chamomile looks much like its cousin, Roman chamomile (*Chamaemelum nobile*), but German chamomile is an annual and must be grown from seed each spring. Roman chamomile may spread to form a lush mat, which can be mowed regularly. Both chamomile species are native to Europe, Africa, and Asia and have become naturalized in North America. Chamomile is widely cultivated. There are other species of chamomile, including several that are indigenous to North America.

Ease of care: Moderate

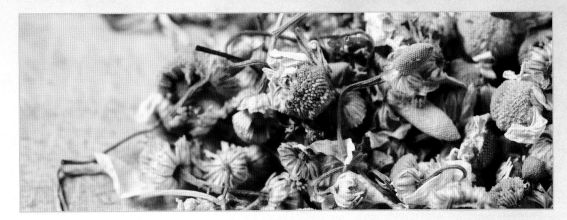

Cultivation: Chamomile grows in full sun, in average to poor, light, dry soil. Plant several chamomiles; single plants are too small to have any impact in a garden.

Propagation: Sow seed in early spring; divide in the spring or fall.

Uses: Chamomile is one of the world's best-loved herbs. The herb produces a pleasant-tasting tea, which has a strong aroma of apples. The early Egyptians valued chamomile and used it to cure malaria and bring down fevers. The ancient Greeks called on chamomile to relieve headaches and treat illnesses of the kidney, liver, and bladder. Today herbalists prescribe the herb to calm nerves and settle upset stomachs, among its other uses.

Chamomile's medicinal properties derive from its essential oils. The herb has three primary medicinal uses: an anti-inflammatory to reduce swelling and infection; an antispasmodic to relieve digestive upsets, headaches, and menstrual cramps; and an anti-infective for cleansing wounds. Chamomile is often found in creams and lotions to soothe sensitive or irritated skin and treat rashes and skin allergies. Cosmetics employ it to reduce puffiness, especially around the eyes. It reduces the swelling that results from allergies or colds. It is used on bruises, sprains, and varicose veins and almost any time the skin becomes inflamed. Chamomile infusions make excellent skin cleansers. Use chamomile both internally and topically to relieve muscle pain. Its calming action not only relieves pain but also induces sleep and relieves nervous indigestion—it has been used to calm children and babies for hundreds of years. Chamomile reduces gastric acid, which helps prevent or speed healing of ulcers. It even shows immune-system activity. Chamomile's fragrant aroma makes it a good addition to potpourri and flower arrangements.

Drink as much chamomile tea as you wish. Use up to 11/2 teaspoons (6 droppers full) of tincture a day. You can also take chamomile as pills, or use it in a vinegar or skin cream. Use a chamomile compress, poultice, or tincture on bruises and inflammation. Add a few drops of essential oil to creams, lotions, or a bath.

Chamomile flowers may cause symptoms of allergies in some people allergic to ragweed and related plants, although the risk of this is quite low.

Part used: Flowers

Preservation: Harvest flowers when fully open. Hang-dry plants; screen-dry flowers.

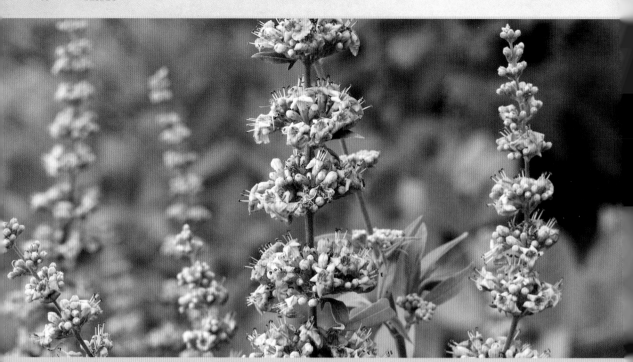

Chaste Tree

Perennial

Botanical Name: *Vitex agnus castus*

Family: Verbenaceae

Height: To 20 ft.

Spread: 6 ft.

Description: Chaste tree is a small tree, with opposite leaves divided into lanceolate leaflets. Its small flowers are lavender or lilac. Native to southern Europe, the herb has been naturalized in warm regions.

Ease of care: Easy

During the Middle Ages, monks used chaste tree to diminish their sexual drive, hence the herb's common name, monk's pepper.

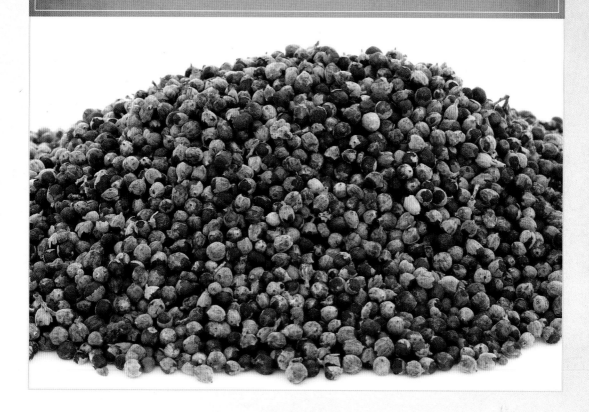

Cultivation: Chaste tree likes sandy or loamy, well-drained soil and full sun.

Propagation: Sow seed in spring; layer or take young woody cuttings in spring.

Uses: Chaste tree, which is often referred to as Vitex, is used primarily to treat women's discomforts. The flavonoids in chaste tree produce a progesterone-like effect. The herb may raise progesterone levels by acting on the brain. Chaste tree helps to normalize and regulate menstrual cycles, reduce premenstrual fluid retention, reduce some cases of acne that may flare up during PMS or menstruation, reduce hot flashes, and treat menopausal bleeding irregularities and other menopausal symptoms. It is also useful in helping dissolve fibroids and cysts in the reproductive system and may be used for treating some types of infertility.

Chaste tree has been used after childbirth to promote milk production. It is a slow-acting herb and may take months to take effect. Because of its complex hormonal actions, be cautious using chaste tree during pregnancy. It may also interfere with hormonal drugs. Little information is available about the physiologic activity of chaste tree in men.

Part used: Berries

Preservation: Gather berries after they ripen; dry or tincture.

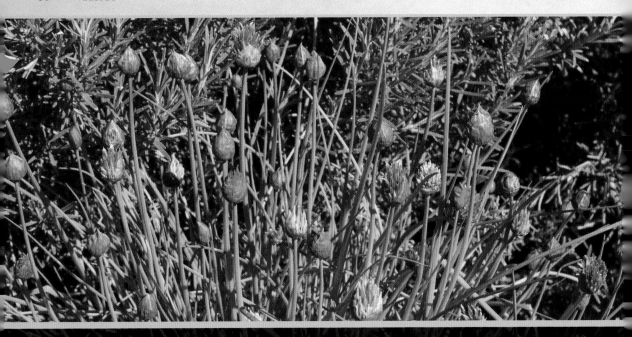

Chives

Perennial

Botanical Name: *Allium schoenoprasum*

Family: Liliaceae

Height: 8–12 in.

Spread: 8 in.

Description: Chives produces clumps of thin leaves that resemble those of onion in appearance and taste. The herb produces abundant, small, rose-purple, globe-shaped flower heads in early summer. Chives may be grown alone or with other plants in containers. The herb is native to Greece, Sweden, the Alps, and parts of northern Great Britain.

Ease of care: Easy

Cultivation: Chives prefers an average to rich soil but manages in almost any soil. The herb grows best in full sun to partial shade. Chives makes a good ornamental plant in the garden. Chives may also be grown as a potted plant indoors at any time of the year. Several new varieties have been developed to produce thicker bunches and longer-lasting flowers. Chives is said to complement growth of carrots, grapes, roses, and tomatoes. The herb deters Japanese beetles and may prevent companion plants from developing black spot, scab, and mildew.

Propagation: Sow seed or divide at any time during the growing season.

Uses: Archaeologists tell us that chives has been in use for at least 5,000 years. By the 16th century, it was a popular European garden herb. Chives' few medicinal properties derive from the sulfur-rich oil found in all members of the onion family. The oil is antiseptic and may help lower blood pressure, but it must be consumed in fairly large quantities. Chives' pleasant taste—like that of mild, sweet onions—complements the flavor of most foods. Use fresh minced leaves in dishes containing potatoes, artichokes, asparagus, cauliflower, corn, tomatoes, peas, carrots, spinach, poultry, fish, veal, cheese, eggs, and, of course, in cream cheese atop your bagel or in sour cream on a baked potato. Add chives at the last minute for best flavor. Flowers are good additions to salads and may be preserved in vinegars.

Part used: Leaves, flowers

Preservation: Harvest leaves any time by trimming off the top one third. Mince leaves and freeze them to obtain full flavor since they do not dry well. Or dry them in the refrigerator to help preserve their color and taste. (Commercial chives are freeze-dried.) Pick flowers before seeds appear and preserve in vinegar.

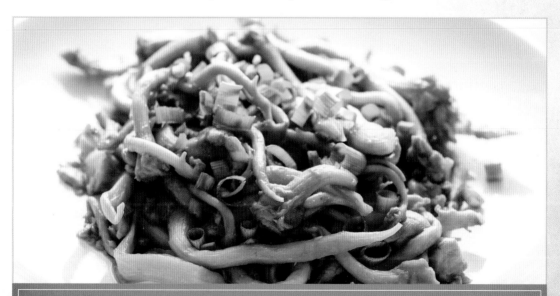

The best way to derive chives' benefits is to add minced leaves liberally to cooked dishes or use a chive vinegar.

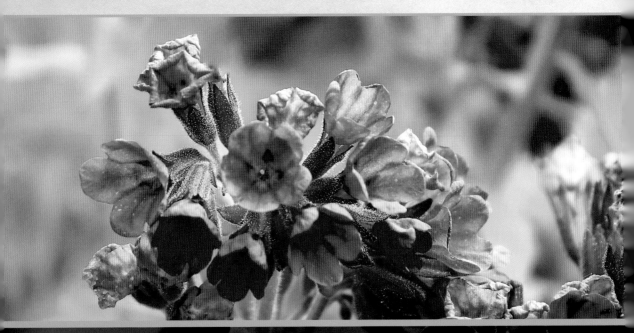

Comfrey

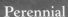

Perennial

Botanical Name: *Symphytum officinale*

Family: Boraginaceae

Height: 3 ft.

Spread: 1 ft.

Description: Comfrey is a hardy, leafy plant that dies down in winter and comes back strong in spring. The herb produces roots that are black outside and white inside and exude a mucilaginous substance when crushed. Various species of comfrey have purple-pink flowers and appear from May through the first frost. The herb is native to Europe and Asia and has become naturalized on every continent. Comfrey is found along stream banks and in moist meadows.

Ease of care: Easy

Cultivation: Comfrey prefers rich to average soil and full sun or partial shade but will grow almost anywhere. The herb is easy to grow, but it is very invasive and difficult to eradicate, so plant it where you can contain it. Once established, comfrey requires little maintenance, but you will have it there forever!

Propagation: Sow seed in spring, divide in fall, take cuttings any time. Set plants 3 feet apart.

Uses: Comfrey has been regarded as a great healer since at least around 400 BC, when the Greeks used it topically to stop bleeding, heal wounds, and mend broken bones. The Romans made comfrey poultices and teas to treat bruises, stomach disorders, and diarrhea. Today herbalists continue to prescribe comfrey for bruises, wounds, and sores. Allantoin, a compound found in comfrey, causes cells to divide and grow, spurring wounds to heal faster. It also inhibits inflammation of the stomach's lining. Comfrey has been recommended for treating bronchitis, asthma, respiratory irritation, peptic ulcers, and stomach and intestinal inflammation. Studies show it inhibits prostaglandins, substances that cause inflammation. It was once promoted as a salad green and potherb; however, internal use of comfrey has become a much-debated topic.

In cosmetic use, comfrey soothes and softens skin and promotes growth of new cells. Comfrey is found in creams, lotions, and bath preparations. It dyes wool brown.

Part used: Root, leaves

Preservation: Dig comfrey roots in late summer or fall.

Precautions: There is some evidence that excessive consumption of comfrey root, especially *Symphytum uplandicum*, may lead to liver damage. It has been suggested that other substances they took simultaneously may have interacted adversely with the comfrey. Comfrey contains pyrrolizidine alkaloids, which are responsible for its harmful effects. The dried leaf contains no pyrrolizidine alkaloids; it is considered relatively safe to use as tea and does contain some of the healing allantoin. The fresh leaves contain very little pyrrolizidine, especially the large, mature leaves.

If using dried root, chop or grind it and dissolve it in hot water to release mucilage for external use. Don't boil comfrey or you'll break down the healing allantoin. You'll notice that most skin salves contain comfrey, so add comfrey root or leaves to oils, salves, and lotions. You can apply a poultice of grated comfrey root or a compress cloth soaked in comfrey tea to sunburns and other skin irritations.

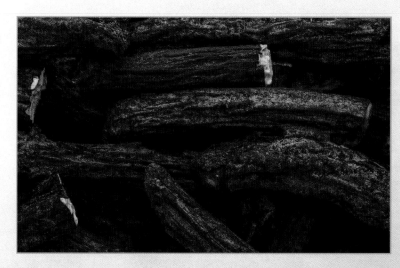

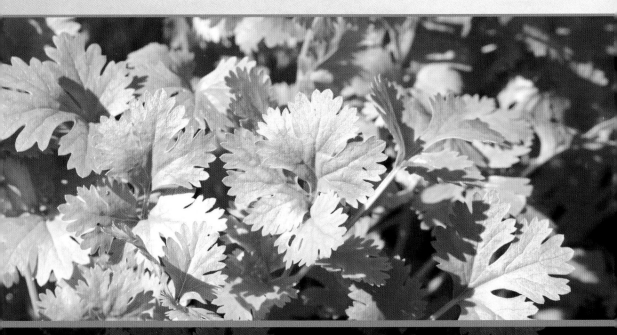

Coriander

Annual

Botanical Name: *Coriandrum sativum*

Family: Apiaceae (Umbelliferae)

Height: 2–3 ft.

Spread: 6 in.

Description: Coriander's bright green, lacy leaves resemble those of flat-leaved Italian parsley when they first spring up from seed, but they become more fernlike as the plant matures. Coriander, also called cilantro and Chinese parsley, flowers from middle to late summer. The herb is native to the eastern Mediterranean region and southern Europe. It is widely cultivated in Morocco, Mexico, Argentina, Canada, India, and the United States, especially in South Carolina.

Ease of care: Easy

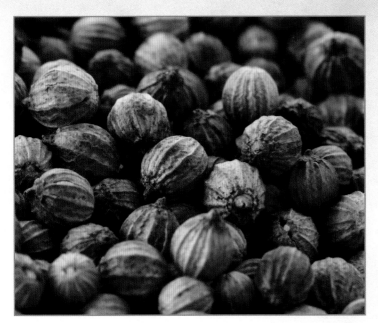

Cultivation: Coriander prefers average, well-drained soil in full sun. Protect fragile stalks from wind. Coriander may enhance growth of anise.

Propagation: Sow seed in spring after soil is warm.

Uses: Coriander has been cultivated for 3,000 years. The Hebrews, who used coriander seed as one of their Passover herbs, probably learned about it from the ancient Egyptians, who revered the plant. The Romans and Greeks used coriander for medicinal purposes and as a spice and preservative. The Chinese believed coriander could make a human immortal. Throughout northern Europe, people would suck on candy-coated coriander seeds when they had indigestion; chewing the seeds soothes an upset stomach, relieves flatulence, aids digestion, and improves appetite. Poultices of coriander seeds have been used to relieve the pain of rheumatism. The Chinese prescribe the tea to treat dysentery and measles. Coriander relieves inflammation and headaches. But its most popular medicinal use has been to flavor strong-tasting medicines and to prevent intestinal gripping common with some laxative formulas.

Coriander's leaf flavor is a cross between sage and citrus. The herb's bold flavor is common to several ethnic cuisines, notably those of China, southeast Asia, Mexico, East India, Spain, Central Africa, and Central and South America. Add young leaves to beets, onions, salads, sausage, clams, oysters, and potatoes. Add seeds to marinades, salad dressings, cheese, eggs, and pickling brines. Coriander seed is used commercially to flavor sugared confections, liqueurs such as Benedictine and Chartreuse, and gin. Its essential oil is found in perfumes, aftershaves, and cosmetics because of its delightfully spicy scent. It is no longer as popular a cosmetic as it was from the 14th to 17th centuries, but coriander "refines" the complexion and was in the famous Eau de Carnes and Carmelite water. It is still used in soaps and deodorants.

Very large doses are reputedly narcotic, but it is unlikely you could eat the quantity needed to produce this effect. Coriander leaves and seeds are almost exclusively eaten, although occasionally the seed is used to flavor medicine.

Part used: Young leaves, seeds

Preservation: Harvest only fresh, young leaves, and freeze them promptly or preserve them in vinegar. Harvest seeds when they start to turn brown. Cut a whole plant and hang-dry upside down inside paper bags to catch seeds.

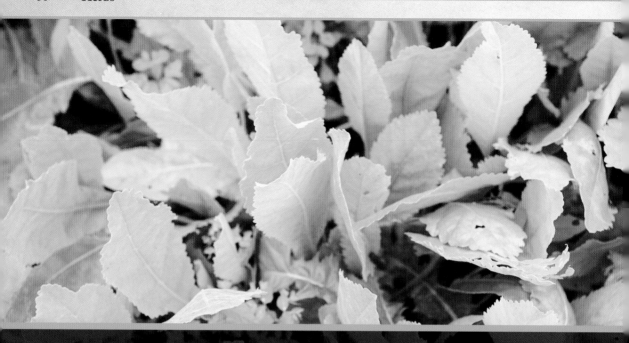

Costmary

Perennial

Botanical Name: *Chrysanthemum balsamita*

Family: Asteraceae (Compositae)

Height: 2 1/2–3 ft.

Spread: 2 ft.

Description: Costmary produces basal clusters of elongated oval leaves. The herb sends up tall flower stems that produce clusters of unremarkable blooms. When leaves are young and fresh, they smell spicy; the scent changes to balsam when the leaves are dried. The herb is native to western Asia. Although it's rarely found growing in the wild, it is cultivated throughout Europe and North America.

Ease of care: Easy

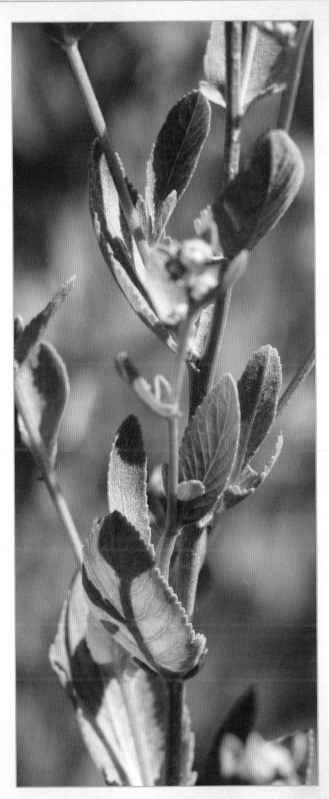

Cultivation: Costmary prefers fertile, well-drained soil in full sun to partial shade.

Propagation: Divide as needed and every few years as clumps become large.

Uses: Costmary flourished in English gardens and was used to spice ale. The herb is antiseptic and slightly astringent and has been used in salves to heal dry, itchy skin. It promotes urine flow and brings down fevers. Although rarely used for this purpose today, its principle medicinal use was as a digestive aid and to treat dysentery, for which it was included in the *British Pharmacopoeia*. The cosmetic water was commonly used to improve the complexion and as a hair rinse. Costmary is good for acne and oily skin and hair.

Costmary's flavor complements beverages, chilled soups, and fruit salads. You can add dried leaves to potpourri, sachets, and baths, or slip them in books to deter bugs that eat paper—this was once a common practice. Dried branches have been used to make herbal baskets.

Costmary is rarely used medicinally, but you could make a tea of the leaves. However, the tea tastes bitter, so add sweeter herbs such as lemon balm and mint.

Part used: Leaves

Preservation: Pick leaves any time. Hang-dry to preserve. Dried costmary retains its scent for a long time.

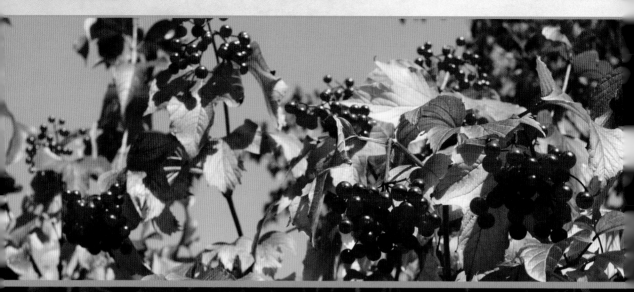

Cramp Bark

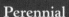

Perennial

Botanical Name: *Viburnum opulus*

Family: Caprifoliaceae

Height: To 13 ft.

Spread: 6 ft.

Description: A relative of black haw and sloe, cramp bark was introduced to England in the 16th century from Holland, where it is known as guelder rose. Also called highbush cranberry or snowball tree, cramp bark has multiple branches that produce three to five lobed, shiny leaves. White flowers appear from early to middle summer, followed by scarlet berries that eventually turn purple. The tree is native to Europe, North Africa, and northern Asia and has become naturalized elsewhere, particularly in Canada and the northern United States. Cramp bark may be found in woodland clearings in wet, loamy soil.

Ease of care: Easy, once established

Cultivation: Cramp bark likes moist, average to rich soil and full sun.

Propagation: Cramp bark grows from seed, although seeds need stratification and may take months to germinate. New shrubs also grow from hardwood cuttings. The easiest way to obtain the herb is to buy a plant from the nursery—it is a popular landscape plant.

Uses: Cramp bark's name tells you how the tree is used. American Indian women relied extensively on cramp bark to ease the pain of menstrual cramps and childbirth. An early American formula known as Mother's Cordial was given to women in childbirth. Cramp bark is used to halt contractions during premature labor and prevent miscarriage. It has also been used to prevent uterine hemorrhaging.

An antispasmodic, cramp bark may reduce leg cramps, muscle spasms, and pain from a stiff neck. Nineteenth-century herbalists often prescribed cramp bark as a sedative and muscle relaxant. The herb's medicinal actions may be attributed in part to a bitter called viburnin, as well as valerianic acid (also found in valerian), salicosides (also found in willow bark), and an antispasmodic constituent. Clinical studies indicate cramp bark may be useful in treating cardiovascular problems, reducing blood pressure and heart palpitations, and fighting influenza viruses. Cramp bark is considered an astringent as well.

The tree's cooked berries taste somewhat like cranberries, which is why it is often called cranberry tree or bush. In Scandinavia, liquor is distilled from the fruit. A Russian brandy, *nastoika*, made with the berries is used as a stomach ulcer remedy. From a species that grows in Japan, the Japanese make a vinegar to treat cirrhosis of the liver.

Use under the care of a physician or herbalist during pregnancy. Use cramp bark with herbs such as wild yam and other uterine relaxants in tea, pills, or tinctures. As a general antispasmodic, blend in with sedative herbs such as valerian. Take up to 1 1/2 teaspoons (about 6 droppers full) of tincture or 6 cups of tea a day to relieve muscle spasms.

Part used: Root, bark

Preservation: Dig roots in summer or fall. Peel bark from the root and dry or tincture. Gather trunk bark in April or May, and tincture or dry.

Precautions: Do not eat fresh berries, which contain viburnin and may cause indigestion. The toxicity dissipates when berries are cooked.

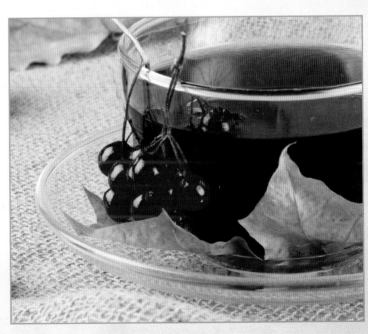

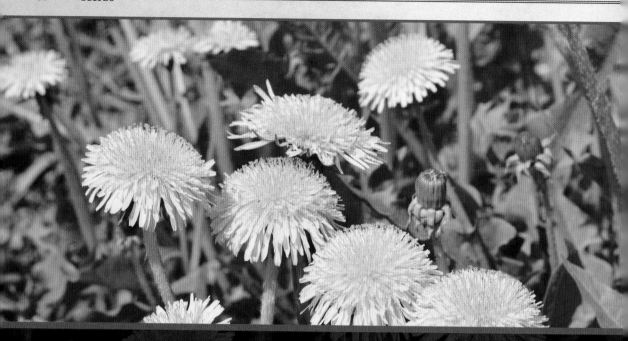

Dandelion

Perennial

Botanical Name: *Taraxacum officinale*

Family: Asteraceae (Compositae)

Height: 6–12 in.

Spread: 1 ft.; may become invasive

Description: Long considered a lawn pest, dandelion produces a taproot that is white on the inside and dark brown on the outside. You're probably familiar with the bright yellow flowers that top dandelion's hollow stems. Flowers appear in late spring and close at night. Dark green leaves are jagged and grow close to the ground in a rosette. Native to Europe and Asia, dandelion has become naturalized throughout temperate regions.

Ease of care: Easy

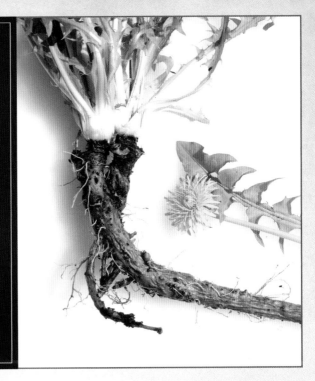

Dandelion root's diuretic properties may help lower blood pressure and relieve premenstrual fluid retention. Unlike most diuretics, it retains potassium rather than flushing it from the body. Clinical studies have favorably compared dandelion's actions with the frequently prescribed diuretic drug Furosemide. Dandelion roots contain inulin and levulin, starchlike substances that are easy to digest, as well as a bitter substance (taraxacin) that stimulates digestion. Dandelion roots, stems, and leaves exude a white sticky resin that dissolves warts, if applied repeatedly.

Cultivation: Dandelion is a wild plant that likes nitrogen-rich soil but will grow just about anywhere. The herb prefers full sun to partial shade. Dandelion is said to enhance growth of fruit trees.

Propagation: Collect seeds from the wild and sow in spring.

Uses: The Arabs were the first to introduce dandelion's healing and nutritive abilities to the Europeans through medical treatises. By the 16th century, dandelion was considered an important culinary and blood-purifying herb in Europe. The root is used to treat liver diseases, such as jaundice and cirrhosis. It also is considered beneficial for building up blood and curing anemia.

Wine made from dandelion flowers tastes like sherry. An Arabian dish, yublo, contains the flower buds and oil, flour, honey, and roses. The roasted ground root makes a good coffee substitute. Dandelion leaves are rich in minerals and vitamins, particularly vitamins A, B2, C, and K and calcium. Add young leaves to salads, or sauté them as you would spinach. The English sometimes put the flowers in sandwiches. Dandelion makes a tonic bath and facial steam. Its flowers produce a yellow dye.

Supplement your diet with fresh dandelion leaves and roots. (The flowers are not usually eaten, but they are used to make wine.) Drink up to 4 to 5 cups a day. Take 1/4 to 1/2 teaspoon tincture (1 to 2 droppers full) up to three times a day.

Part used: Root, leaves, flowers

Preservation: Gather leaves in the spring, flowers in the summer, and roots in the fall.

Precautions: The white latex in fresh dandelion is caustic and may cause skin irritation and digestive disturbances, so dry the root before using.

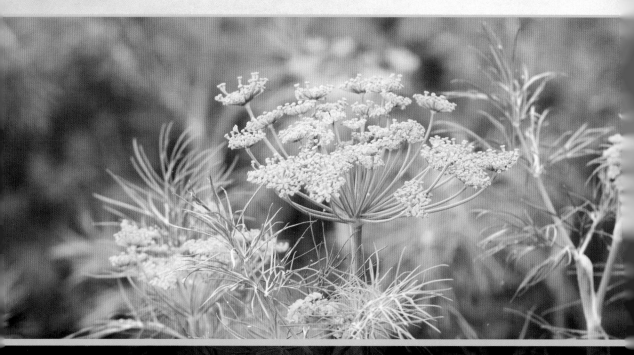

Dill

Annual

Botanical Name: *Anethum graveolens*

Family: Apiaceae (Umbelliferae)

Height: 2–3 ft.

Spread: 6–12 in.

Description: Dill produces fine-cut, fernlike leaves on tall, fragile stems. It is a blue-green annual with attractive yellow flower umbels and yellow-green seed heads. The herb blooms from July through September. Native to the Mediterranean region and southwest Asia, it has become naturalized throughout North America.

Ease of care: Easy

Cultivation: Dill likes light, moist, sandy soil in full sun. Because it does not transplant well, sow in place and thin as needed. Grow dill in clumps or rows, so fragile stems can support each other. Some gardeners believe dill enhances the growth of cabbage, onions, and lettuce.

Propagation: Sow seed in late fall or early spring. Plant at three-week intervals during spring and early summer for a fresh supply all season.

Uses: Dill derives from an old Norse word meaning "to lull," and, indeed, the herb once was used to induce sleep in babies with colic. Herbalists also use dill to relieve gas and to stimulate flow of mother's milk. Dill stimulates the appetite and settles the stomach, but the seeds have also been chewed to lessen the appetite and stop the stomach from rumbling—something that parishioners found useful during all-day church services. In India, it is used to treat ulcers, fevers, uterine pain, and problems with the eyes and kidneys, usually in a formula with other herbs. In Ethiopia, the seeds are chewed to relieve a headache.

Add minced dill leaves to salads and use as a garnish. Seeds go well with fish, lamb, pork, poultry, cheese, cream, eggs, and an array of vegetables, including cabbage, onions, cauliflower, squash, spinach, potatoes, and broccoli. Of course, dill pickles would not be the same without dill seed and weed. The herb is particularly popular in Russia and Scandinavia. Its taste somewhat resembles caraway, which shares a similar chemistry.

By far, the most popular way to use dill is to incorporate it into your food to aid digestion. Although you could use it in an herb tea, sweeter digestive herbs such as anise are preferred. An essential oil is available; however, it is used mostly by the food industry.

Part used: Leaves, seeds

Preservation: Clip fresh leaves as needed. Flavor is best retained for later use if frozen; pick leaves just as flowers begin to open. For seeds, harvest entire plants when seed heads begin to turn brown. Hang-dry upside down in paper bags to catch seeds.

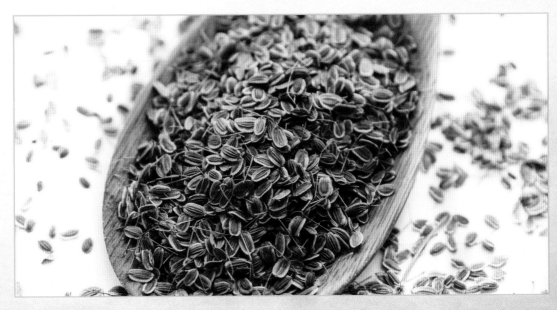

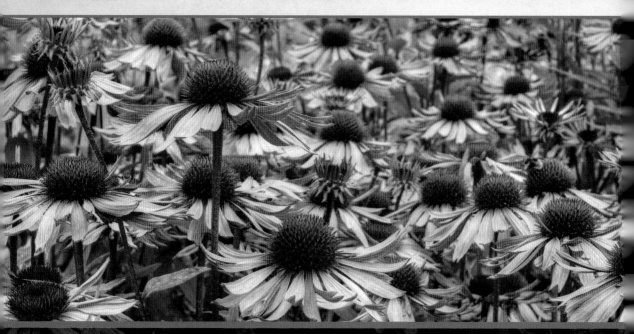

Echinacea

Perennial

Botanical Name: *Echinacea purpurea*

Family: Asteraceae (Compositae)

Height: To 4 ft.

Spread: 2 ft.

Description: Also known as purple coneflower, echinacea resembles the black-eyed Susan. The herb produces long black roots and stout, sturdy stems covered with bristly hairs. Cone-shaped flower heads, which appear from middle to late summer, are composed of numerous tiny purple florets surrounded by deep pink petals. Leaves are pale green to dark green. Echinacea is native to prairies from southern Canada to Texas.

Ease of care: Easy

Cultivation: Echinacea prefers average, well-drained soil and full sun to light shade. The herb may fall prey to leaf spot or Japanese beetles.

Propagation: Sow seed in spring. Mulch in winter. Dig up the plant about every four years, divide, and replant in fertilized soil.

Uses: American Indians used echinacea extensively to treat the bites of snakes and poisonous insects, burns, and wounds; the root facilitates wound healing. (Sometimes the seeds are combined with the roots for medicinal use.) Echinacea is prescribed to treat various infections, mumps, measles, and eczema. A compound in echinacea prevents damage to collagen in the skin and connective tissues when taken internally. Recent studies suggest that, applied topically, echinacea may treat sunburn.

Today, echinacea root is used primarily to boost the immune system and help the body fight disease. Besides bolstering several chemical substances that direct immune response, echinacea increases the number and activity of white blood cells (the body's disease-fighting agents), raises the level of interferon (a substance that enhances immune function), increases production of substances the body produces to fight cancers, and helps remove pollutants from the lungs. Many studies support echinacea's ability to fend off disease.

Another species, *E. angustifolia*, is used interchangeably with *E. purpurea* although the chemistry of the two species is slightly different.

Take capsules, tea, or tinctures. Most herbalists recommend large, frequent doses at the onset of a cold, flu, sinus infection, or other illness. For acute infection, take 1/4 teaspoon (1 dropper full) of tincture every 1 to 3 hours for a day or two, then reduce the dosage. Take echinacea three times a day for several weeks; then abstain for several weeks before using again. Echinacea is often used alone but may be combined with other anti-infection and immune-stimulating herbs.

Part used: Root, seeds, leaves; flowers and seed heads for crafts

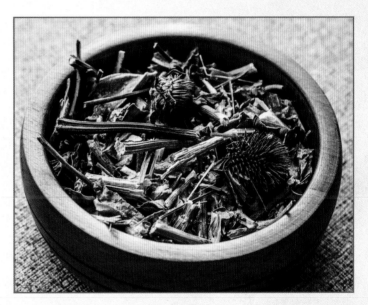

Preservation: Harvest roots after the plant begins to die back in the fall. Replant the crown after you have taken the root. Dry or tincture.

Precautions: Echinacea has been shown to be very nontoxic and safe even for children. Some herbalists believe echinacea should not be used by people with auto-immune disorders such as lupus or rheumatoid arthritis because their immune systems are already overstimulated.

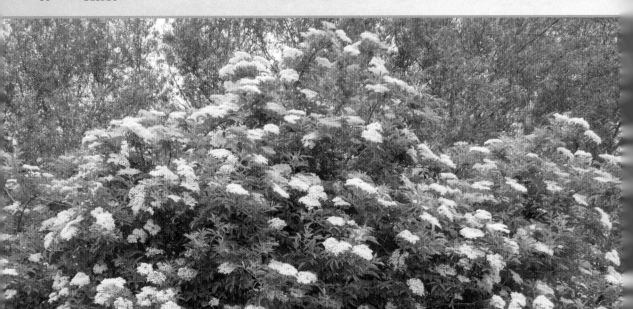

Elderberry

Perennial

Botanical Name: *Sambucus nigra*

Family: Caprifoliaceae

Height: 12–50 ft.

Spread: To 20 ft.; may become invasive

Description: Elderberry comprises about 13 species of deciduous shrubs native to North America and Europe. European settlers brought elderberry plants with them to the American colonies. Its flowers are white and plate-shaped, the leaves are pinnate (resembling a feather) and may be toothed, and its fruit appears in purple-blue clusters.

Ease of care: Easy

Cultivation: Elderberry prefers fertile, moist soil and full sun to partial shade. Propagate the suckers or grow plants from seeds or cuttings. Elderberry may require maintenance since it likes to sprawl.

Uses: Elderberry has probably been used medicinally and nutritively for as long as human beings have gathered plants. Evidence of elderberry plants has been uncovered in Stone Age sites. Ancient people used elderberries to dye their hair black. The wood of old stems is still used to make musical instruments by Native Americans and Europeans.

In the kitchen, the berries are used to make jams, jellies, chutneys, preserves, wines, and teas. For decades, elder flower water was on the dressing tables of proper young ladies who used it to treat sunburn and eradicate freckles. It is still sometimes used in Europe for these purposes. Yellow and violet dyes are made from the leaves and berries, respectively.

Medicinally, elderberry has been used as a mild digestive stimulant and diaphoretic. Elder flowers decrease inflammation, so they are often included in preparations to treat burns and swellings and in cosmetics that reduce puffiness. The berries have been used traditionally in Europe to treat flu, gout, and rheumatism as well as to improve general health. Several tales attribute longevity to the elderberry.

Recent studies in Israel found the berry is a potent antiviral that fights influenza virus B, the cause of one of the common forms of flu. Recognizing that it has long been used as a flu remedy, researchers at the Hebrew University Hadasah Medical Centre in Jerusalem conducted clinical studies and found the berry reduced fever, coughs, and muscle pain within 24 hours. After taking an elderberry syrup only two days, almost two-thirds of those with influenza reported complete recovery. The Centre also found that elderberry stimulates the immune system. The berries are currently under investigation for their ability to inhibit the herpes and Epstein-Barr viruses as well as HIV, the virus that causes AIDS. The berries are also rich in compounds that improve heart and circulatory health.

Drink the flower tea freely. Take up to 3 cups of tea or 1 teaspoon (4 droppers full) of tincture made from the berry. Elderberry is also available in juices.

Part used: Berries, flowers

Preservation: Pick flowers in full bloom. Use them fresh or dried. Harvest berries when juicy and ripe.

Precautions: The elderberry that bears blue fruit is perfectly safe to eat, although large quantities of the raw berries can cause some indigestion and act as a laxative. Cooking the berries before eating them cancels this action. The leaves, bark, and root, on the other hand, are slightly toxic and should not be used internally. Don't use the elder plant that bears red berries: This plant is a different species *(Sambucus pubens)*.

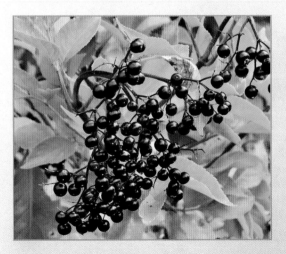

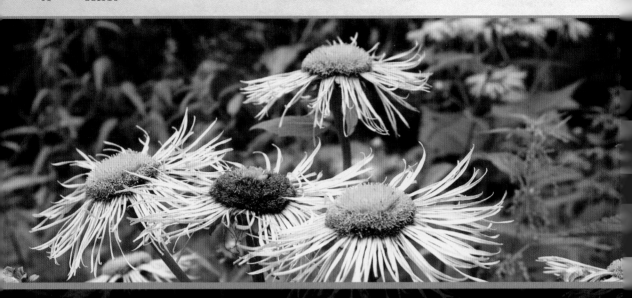

Elecampane

Perennial

Botanical Name: *Inula helenium*

Family: Asteraceae (Compositae)

Height: 4–6 ft.

Spread: 2 ft.

Description: Also known as wild sunflower, velvet dock, scabwort, and horseheal, elecampane is a tall, attractive plant. Sturdy, with a round, coarse, woolly stem, elecampane produces blooms that resemble sunflowers. Elecampane's leaves are toothed and bristly on the upper surface, velvety on the underside. Elecampane ranges from central and southern Europe to northwest Asia. It has been naturalized in many parts of North America—from Nova Scotia to North Carolina and west to Missouri. Often, it's found in damp soil, near ruins, and along roadsides or woodland edges.

Ease of care: Easy

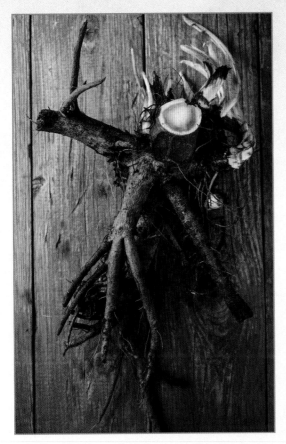

Cultivation: Elecampane likes moist, moderately fertile soil or a well-drained clay loam in full sun to partial shade.

Propagation: Elecampane may be started from seeds sown indoors in late winter and transplanted later. You can also obtain new plants from offshoots or 2-inch root cuttings taken from a mature plant in autumn. Use moist, sandy soil to cover the cuttings, and keep them in a cool room. By early spring, the roots should develop into plants.

Uses: Elecampane's Latin name, *helenium*, refers to the legend that Helen of Troy carried a handful of elecampane on the day Paris abducted her, sparking the Trojan War. Perhaps she carried it because she had worms: Elecampane has been used for centuries to expel parasites in the digestive system, and today we know it contains a compound that expels intestinal worms.

But elecampane has been used most often for treating respiratory diseases. It is especially good for shortness of breath and bronchial problems. Early American colonists grew it for use as an expectorant; in Europe, people with asthma chewed on the root. Indian Ayurvedic physicians prescribe elecampane for chest conditions. In China, the plant is known as hsuan-fu-hua and is used to make syrup, lozenges, and candy to treat bronchitis and asthma.

European studies show that elecampane promotes menstruation and may be useful in reducing blood pressure. The herb also has been shown to have some sedative effect. The root is added to many medicines and used as a flavoring for sweets. Cordials and sugar cakes are still made from it in parts of Europe. You'll find the flower heads in dried craft arrangements.

Take as tea, tincture, or pills. Make into syrup or lozenges for coughs. Elecampane is often mixed with other herbs that are good for the lungs, such as mullein, licorice, and plantain.

Part used: Root

Preservation: Harvest plant roots in the fall of the plant's second year, after it has gone through two hard frosts. Harvest seed heads for crafts.

Precautions: Avoid elecampane if you're pregnant, as the herb has been used traditionally to promote menstruation. Studies have shown that a small dose of elecampane lowers blood sugar levels in animals, but higher doses raise them. Thus, people with diabetes should be careful when using the herb. People occasionally develop a rash from skin contact with the herb.

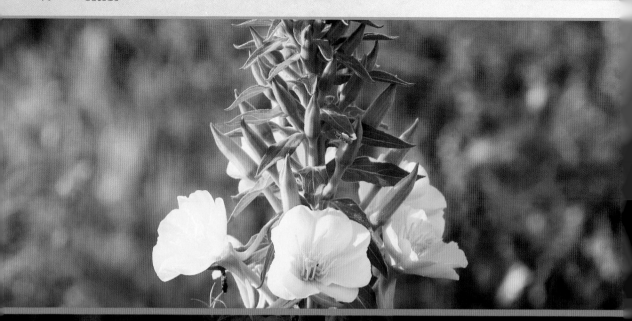

Evening Primrose

Biennial

Botanical Name: *Oenothera biennis*

Family: Onagraceae

Height: 3–6 ft

Spread: 1 1/2 ft.

Description: Some people are so busy during the day they don't have time to enjoy their herb gardens until after the moon rises. If you're one of those folks, evening primrose is the perfect herb for your garden. Its clear yellow flowers unclasp and blossom in the evening. Later in the growing season, evening primrose flowers may remain open during the day. Evening primrose flowers from early summer to mid-autumn. The stem is sturdy, rough, hairy, and reddish; its seeds round, beige, and oily. The plant's leaf is long, oval, and pointed.

Ease of care: Easy

Cultivation: Don't try to grow evening primrose indoors. The plant needs a sunny, open site, with well-drained soil.

Propagation: Sow seeds in spring to early summer; thin to 12 inches by autumn.

Uses: The boiled root of evening primrose, which tastes something like a sweet parsnip, may be pickled or tossed raw in salads. The plant once was grown in monasteries; more recently scientists have found that the seeds contain a rare substance called gamma-linoleic acid (better known as GLA), which may have value in treating multiple sclerosis, thrombosis, premenstrual symptoms, menopausal discomfort, alcohol withdrawal, hyperactivity, and psoriasis. In one study, more than half the study participants found that their PMS symptoms completely disappeared when they used evening primrose. In another study, more than half the arthritis patients who took evening primrose oil also found relief. The oil, when combined with zinc supplements, improves dry eyes and brittle nails, although it often takes two to three months to notice improvement in these conditions. Leaves and bark have been used to ease cough spasms.

Evening primrose also helps regenerate damaged liver cells. It is thought to prevent liver damage, stop alcohol from impairing brain cells, and lessen the symptoms of a hangover.

Part used: Seed, leaves, stems

Preservation: Wait two years to dig up the roots.

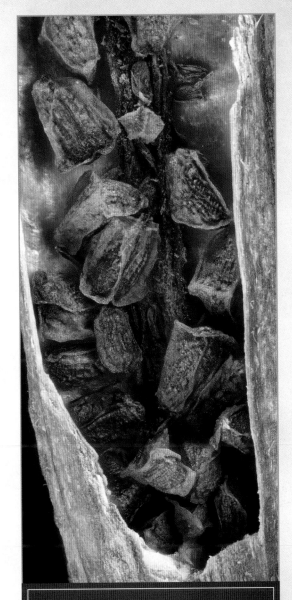

Purchase oil of evening primrose in capsules and follow package directions. The capsules are expensive, but many people find they can reduce the recommended dose after a period of use. Unfortunately, the oil cannot be obtained from the seeds at home—a special process is required to extract it.

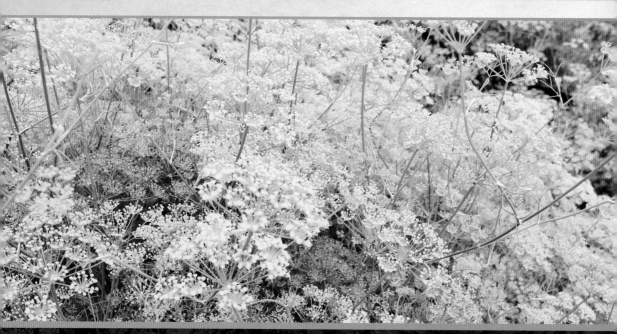

Fennel

Perennial

Botanical Name: *Foeniculum vulgare*

Family: Apiaceae (Umbelliferae)

Height: 4–7 ft.

Spread: 3 ft.

Description: With its feathery leaves, fennel looks much like a large version of its relative, dill. This fairly hardy perennial flowers from June through October. Sweet fennel *(F. vulgare dulce)*, the variety sold in grocery stores, produces celery-like stalks known as *finochhio*. Both varieties taste similar to anise or licorice. Fennel is native to the Mediterranean region and widely naturalized elsewhere. It loves to grow by the ocean and near streams.

Ease of care: Easy

Cultivation: Fennel likes alkaline soil; you can add lime if soil is very acidic, although the herb is not fussy. Grow in full sun to partial shade in well-drained, average soil. Shelter fennel from heavy winds because the plant's fragile stems blow over easily.

Propagation: Sow seeds in late fall or early spring.

Uses: The Greeks gave fennel to nursing mothers to increase milk flow. Early physicians also considered fennel a remedy for poor eyesight, weight loss, hiccups, nausea, gout, and many other illnesses. Fennel is a carminative (relieves gas and pain in the bowels), weak diuretic, and mild digestive stimulant. Herbalists often recommend fennel tea to soothe an upset stomach and dispel gas. It aids digestion, especially of fat. In Europe, a popular children's carminative is still made with fennel, chamomile, caraway, coriander, and bitter orange peel. Fennel is also a urinary tract tonic that lessens inflammation and helps eliminate kidney stones.

Fennel tastes like a more bitter version of anise. Use leaves in salads and as garnishes. You can eat tender stems as you would celery, and add seeds to desserts, breads, cakes, cookies, and beverages. Mince bulbs of sweet fennel and eat raw or braise. Fennel complements fish, sausage, duck, barley, rice, cabbage, beets, pickles, potatoes, lentils, breads, and eggs. Add it to butters, cheese spreads, and salad dressings. Fennel essential oil is found commercially in condiments, liqueurs, and aromatherapy cosmetics such as creams, perfumes, and soaps. It has a reputation for improving the complexion and decreasing wrinkles. A fennel infusion acts as a skin cleanser and antiseptic. It reduces bruising when applied topically. The herb dyes wool shades of yellow and brown.

Use fennel in food and herb teas. It is sometimes used in formulas to treat digestion or urinary tract problems. Laxative formulas may use fennel to ease the activity of the intestines and reduce gas and bloating. Make a facial cream with fennel seeds, lavender, and rosemary.

Part used: Leaves, seeds

Preservation: Snip leaves any time to use fresh, or freeze. Harvest whole plants just before they bloom, and hang to dry. To harvest seeds, cut down plants when seeds turn brown. Hang-dry in paper bags to catch seeds.

Precautions: Fennel has mild estrogenic properties, so avoid it if you're pregnant. Very large amounts can overstimulate the nervous system. Be especially careful using the essential oil.

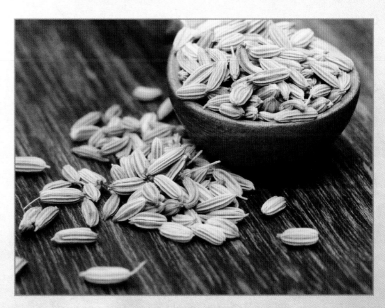

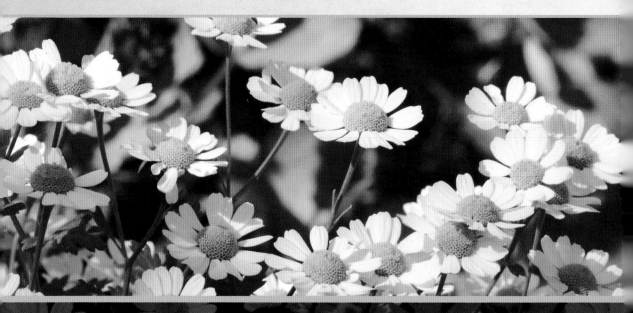

Feverfew

Perennial or Biennial

Botanical Name: *Tanacetum parthenium*
(formerly *Chrysanthemum parthenium*)

Family: Asteraceae (Compositae)

Height: To 2 ft.

Spread: 1–2 ft., spreading

Description: Feverfew is an erect herb that produces a branched root and many stems. Its multiple flowers are small and white, with yellow centers, like its cousin, the daisy, and it looks somewhat like chamomile. Flowers appear from midsummer through fall. Feverfew's leaves are yellowish green with a bitter scent. The herb is native to central and southern Europe and has become naturalized throughout temperate regions, including North and South America. Feverfew reportedly grew abundantly around the Parthenon in Athens; hence its botanical name *parthenium*.

Ease of care: Easy

Cultivation: Feverfew prefers average, well-drained soil and full sun to partial shade.

Propagation: Sow seeds or divide roots in spring. Take cuttings in fall or spring.

Uses: Feverfew's common name derives from the Latin *febrifugia*, which means "driver out of fevers." The Romans used the herb extensively for this purpose, and the Greeks employed it to normalize irregular contractions in childbirth. Today feverfew leaves are best known for their ability to fight headaches, particularly migraines. The herb's constituents relax blood vessels in the brain and inhibit secretion of substances that cause pain. Feverfew is most effective when used long-term to prevent chronic migraines, but some people find it helpful when taken at the onset of a headache. When patients at the Department of Medicine and Haemotology in Nottingham, England, ate fresh feverfew leaves for three months, they had fewer migraines and less nausea when they did experience one. Their blood pressure was reduced, and they reported feelings of well-being. Feverfew also is reported to reduce inflammation in joints and tissues. It has been prescribed for treating menstrual cramps.

Pyrethrin, an active ingredient, is a potent insect repellent. Feverfew's leaves and stems produce a dye that is greenish-yellow.

The best way to take feverfew for migraines is to eat three or four leaves a day. Be forewarned that the leaves are bitter. If raw leaves irritate your mouth, are too bitter, or are unavailable, take 1 to 3 capsules (preferably with freeze-dried feverfew) or 1/2 to 1 teaspoon (2 to 4 droppers full) of tincture daily. Commercial preparations are usually made from leaves but may also contain flowers. Drink up to 3 cups of tea a day. Combine with other, more palatable, herbs, such as mint, to improve the taste. Recent studies show that the flowers are also effective medicinally.

Part used: Leaves, flowers

Preservation: The best time to gather leaves is just before flowering, but you can harvest them throughout the summer. Tincture to retain the maximum amount of medicine.

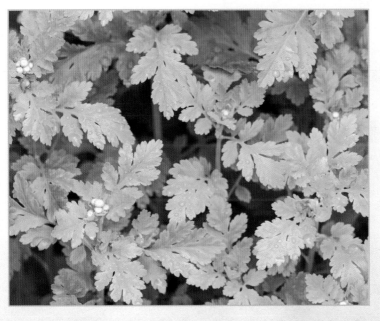

Precautions: Feverfew may cause stomach upset. Chewing raw leaves regularly may irritate the mouth. Tinctures and capsules do not cause such irritation. Because feverfew relaxes blood vessels, it may increase blood flow during menstruation. Some people develop allergic reactions after prolonged exposure to it.

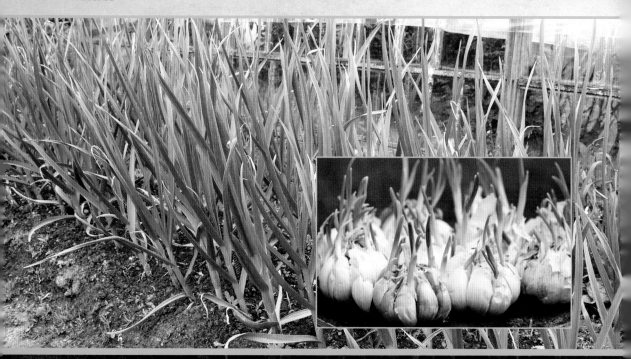

Garlic

Perennial or Biennial

Botanical Name: *Allium sativum*

Family: Liliacea

Height: To 2 ft.

Spread: 6 in.

Description: Garlic produces a compound bulb composed of numerous cloves encased in a papery sheath. Flowers are small and white to pinkish. Long, slender green leaves arise from the bulb. The herb may have originated in southern Siberia; it is cultivated extensively around the world.

Ease of care: Easy

Cultivation: Garlic likes rich, deep, well-drained soil and full sun. Garlic contains fungicides and is thought to repel pests from companion plants.

Propagation: Sow seeds in the fall or plant cloves in early spring for a midsummer harvest. Plant cloves with the pointed side up.

Uses: Garlic has been prized for millennia, used by the Egyptians, Hebrews, Romans, Greeks, and Chinese. Garlic is one of the most extensively researched and widely used plants. Its actions are diverse and affect nearly every body system. The herb boasts antibiotic, antifungal, and antiviral properties and is reported to be effective against many influenza strains, as well as herpes simplex type I. During World War I, field physicians applied garlic juice to infected wounds. Allicin, which gives garlic its distinctive odor, is as effective as a 1 percent penicillin solution in destroying bacteria, fungi, and yeast.

Garlic has been used to treat streptococcal infections, dysentery, whooping cough, and even tuberculosis. Several of garlic's sulfur compounds are noxious to parasites. Garlic inhibits blood clotting and keeps platelets from clumping, which improves blood flow and reduces the risk of stroke. It reduces cholesterol levels, making it a preventive for heart diseases. One study found that people who regularly ate garlic had almost half as many heart attacks. Garlic lowers blood pressure by relaxing the vein and artery walls, keeping them open to improve blood flow. Constituents in garlic appear to increase insulin levels and lower high blood sugar levels. Chinese scientists are investigating garlic's potential as a preventive treatment for stomach cancer. And a University of Minnesota study

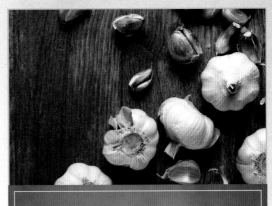

One of the best ways to consume garlic is to eat it raw. When cooked, the stronger the flavor is, the more medicinal value it has. You can also take 1 to 2 capsules of garlic two to three times a day. Take 1/4 teaspoon (1 dropper full) of garlic tincture in a glass of water, two to four times a day. A good antifungal treatment is to use garlic vinegar (garlic tincture made with vinegar).

suggests that women who eat garlic may lower their risk of colon cancer.

Garlic's strong oniony taste has endeared it to cooks all over the world. You may add garlic to butters, cheese spreads, breads, all sorts of vegetables, stuffings, sauces, marinades, salad dressings, stews, soups, and meat dishes. Dried flower heads make an interesting addition to floral arrangements.

Part used: Cloves

Preservation: Harvest garlic when tops turn brown in midsummer; dry in a cool, dark spot.

Precautions: Some people who consume large amounts of garlic feel nauseous or hot or have gas and bloating. Garlic juice may irritate the skin or mucous membranes of sensitive people.

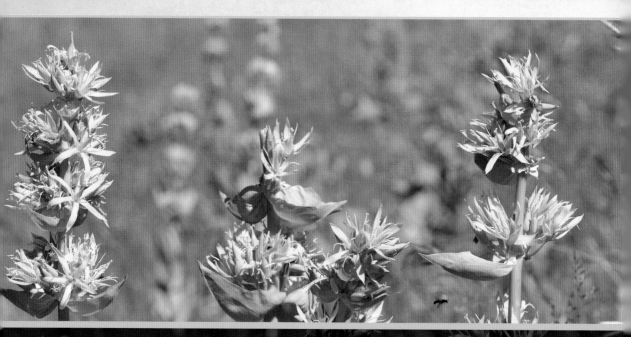

Gentian

Perennial

Botanical Name: *Gentiana lutea*

Family: Gentianaceae

Height: To 3 ft.; occasionally taller

Spread: 1 ft.

Description: Also called bitter root, gentian produces an interesting-looking root that may grow 1 to 2 feet long and 1 to 2 inches thick. Fresh roots are pale yellow; roots have a strong, perhaps disagreeable odor and are extremely bitter. Gentian's leaves, found at each stem joint, are smooth, waxy, and oval and light to medium green. The herb produces abundant, oblong fruit capsules.

Ease of care: Moderate

Cultivation: Gentian likes neutral to acid soil that is moist and well drained. The plant requires partial shade. Once satisfactorily transplanted, the plants require little attention. But they need abundant moisture and shelter from cold, dry winds and direct sunshine. Once a year, refresh the bed with acid soil or peat moss. If the temperature in your area dips well below freezing, mulch gentian with hay or evergreen boughs to protect it.

Propagation: It's possible, though difficult, to grow gentian from seeds, which require frost or stratification to germinate. Even then, they may take up to a year to produce seedlings. For most gardeners, the best bet is to start gentian plants from crown divisions or transplanted roots.

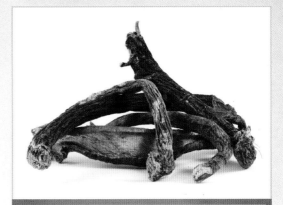

To make gentian bitters, infuse 3 ounces of chopped gentian root in 1 pint of brandy and strain after two weeks. Dilute with water before taking. Take 1/4 to 1 teaspoon at a time.

Uses: Gentian root has been prized as a digestive bitter for more than 3,000 years—the Egyptians, Arabs, Greeks, and Romans used it. In India, Ayurvedic doctors used gentian to treat fevers, venereal disease, jaundice, and other illnesses of the liver. Colonists in Virginia and the Carolinas discovered Indians using a gentian decoction to treat back pain. Chinese physicians use it to treat digestive disorders, sore throat, headache, and arthritis. Gentian, moreover, has been used to increase menstruation, thus easing painful periods.

Today, gentian is used commercially to make liqueurs, vermouth, digestive bitters, and aperitifs. The herb's bitterness increases gastric secretions and helps a sluggish appetite or poor digestion. It is especially useful for problems digesting fat or protein. Researchers in Germany found that it cures heartburn, intestinal inflammation, and general indigestion. It also destroys several types of intestinal worms.

Gentian is rarely made into tea because it is so bitter. If you use gentian tincture, take 1/4 to 1 teaspoon (1 to 4 droppers full) diluted in a small amount of water, 30 minutes before meals.

Part used: Root; flowers in dried arrangements

Preservation: Dig up gentian roots in late summer or autumn, then dry them slowly to cure them. Harvest flowers as soon as they bloom, and dry them for use in decorations.

Precautions: Don't take gentian if you are pregnant. Although no studies have shown it is dangerous, gentian has been used to promote menstruation. Gentian also contains constituents that may elevate blood pressure. Although the Food and Drug Administration has approved gentian for use in foods and alcoholic beverages, large doses may cause nausea and vomiting. The gentian violet sold in pharmacies is not made from gentian: It is a very potent chemical used to treat skin infection.

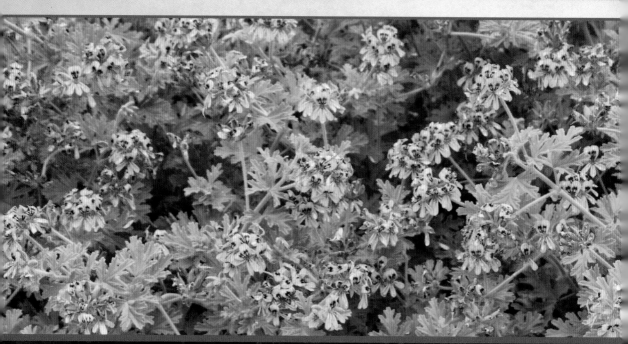

Geranium, Scented

Perennial

Botanical Name: *Pelargonium graveolens*

Family: Geraniaceae

Height: 2 ft.

Spread: 1 ft.

Description: Botanically, these fragrant plants are not really geraniums, but pelargoniums. The leaves are frilly, soft, and well-veined; if you rub against them they emit a distinctive fragrance. The flowers are pink and unscented. The leaves of the different species come in a variety of shapes and sizes. Native to South Africa, the scented geranium has become naturalized in the eastern Mediterranean region, India, Australia, and New Zealand. The plant is widely cultivated.

Ease of care: Moderate

Cultivation: A tender plant, the scented geranium will not tolerate freezing temperatures. It needs rich, dry, loamy, well-drained soil and light shade.

Propagation: The plants are best started from cuttings in spring or summer and transplanted after two to three weeks.

Uses: You could call the scented geranium the potpourri plant. The herb comes in a wide variety of fragrances, including rose, apple, lemon, lime, apricot, strawberry, coconut, and peppermint, making it an ideal addition to potpourri and sachets. The plant was considered fashionable in Colonial and Victorian times.

Herbalists sometimes recommend the astringent herb for treating diarrhea and ulcers and to stop bleeding. The essential oil is used to treat ringworm, lice, shingles, and herpes. The pharmaceutical industry uses one of the antiseptic compounds in geranium called geraniol. The leaves of some varieties, including rose, may be used to flavor cookies and jelly. Add other leaves, such as peppermint, to herbal teas. Added to facial steams and baths, they are cleansing and healing to the skin. The scent is popular in men's products—it blends well with woodsy and citrus fragrances. Rose geranium is used in many aromatherapy products for its relaxing and emotional balancing properties. This species is also added to cosmetics to improve the complexion.

Scented geranium is used most often as an essential oil. Dilute the essential oil in vegetable oil, lotion, or cream for skin care, as a topical medicine, or as a cosmetic. Use the leaves in cooking or to make flavored herb tea.

Part used: Leaves

Preservation: Gather leaves at any time and use fresh or dry. Gather flowers as soon as they bloom.

The fresh leaves of scented geranium can be added to jellies and fruit dishes or placed on desserts. For a unique herbal treat, place the leaves in the bottom of a buttered cake pan before pouring in the batter. When you turn the finished cake over, it will be decorated with the herb leaves.

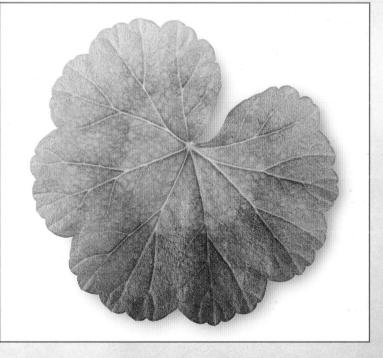

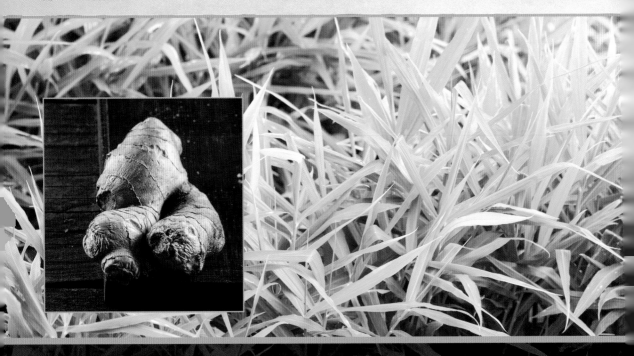

Ginger

Perennial

Botanical Name: *Zingiber officinale*

Family: Zingiberaceae

Height: 1–4 ft.

Spread: 1 1/2 ft.

Description: This tropical, aromatic herb produces a knotty, buff-colored tuberous rhizome. Leaves are grasslike, and flowers are dense, conelike, greenish-purple spikes with edging. Native to southeast Asia, ginger is cultivated elsewhere, including south Florida.

Ease of care: Easy

Cultivation: Ginger requires fertile, moist, well-drained soil and full sun to partial shade. The plant thrives in hot, humid climates, making it suitable for gardens in parts of the American South. Elsewhere, grow ginger in a greenhouse or indoors in a container.

Propagation: Purchase green roots from a nursery or grocery store and plant the "eyes" in loam, sand, peat moss, and compost.

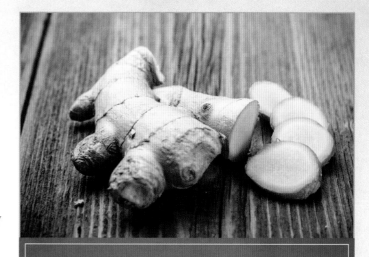

Take up to 6 cups of tea or 11/2 teaspoons tincture (6 droppers full) a day. For nausea, take 1 to 2 ginger capsules every 2 to 6 hours. Grate ginger root for a poultice. Ginger is often added to other herb formulas both for its taste and versatile medicinal uses. Ginger is also medicinal when added to foods.

Uses: Most every child knows the taste of ginger. It's the prime ingredient in ginger ale, gingerbread, and gingersnaps. But the popular kitchen spice enjoys a rich history as a medicinal herb as well. Ginger is a potent anti-nausea medication, useful for treating morning sickness, motion sickness, and nausea accompanying gastroenteritis (stomach "flu"). As a stomach calming aid, ginger reduces gas, bloating, and indigestion and aids in the body's absorption of nutrients and other herbs. Ginger is also a valuable deterrent to several types of intestinal worms. And the herb may work as a therapy and preventive treatment for some migraine headaches and rheumatoid arthritis.

Ginger promotes perspiration if ingested in large amounts. Use internally or topically. The herb stimulates circulation, so if you are cold, you can use warm ginger tea to help raise your body heat. Ginger may occasionally promote menstrual flow. It also prevents platelets from clumping and thins the blood, which reduces the risk of atherosclerosis and blood clots. Grated ginger poultices or compresses ease lung congestion when placed on the chest and alleviate gas, nausea, and menstrual cramps when laid on the abdomen.

Ginger is a staple of many cuisines, including those of southeast Asia, India, Japan, the Caribbean, and North Africa. Add the spicy chopped root to beverages, fruits, meats, fish, preserves, pickles, and a variety of vegetables. Use ground ginger in breads, cookies, and other desserts.

Part used: Root (rhizome)

Preservation: Pull up ginger 8 to 12 months after you plant it, and remove leafstalks and fibers from the root. Use fresh, or tincture or dry.

Precautions: Although ginger is prescribed for nausea, some people develop this symptom after ingesting very large amounts.

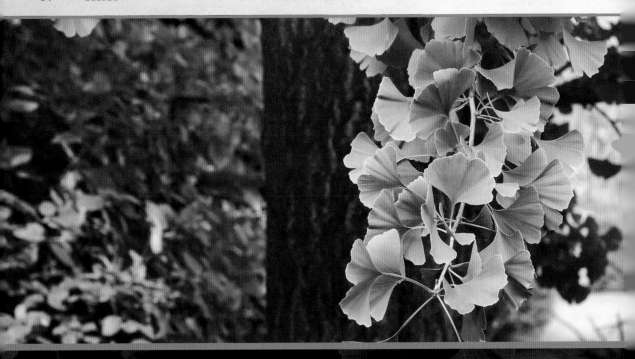

Ginkgo

Perennial

Botanical Name: *Ginkgo biloba*

Family: Ginkgoaceae

Height: To 100 ft.

Spread: 20 ft.

Description: This stately deciduous tree produces male and female flowers on separate plants. Female plants produce orange-yellow fruits the size of large olives. In the fall its leaves turn gold. Found throughout the temperate world, ginkgo may be grown in many parts of the United States. It is cultivated extensively.

Ease of care: Easy

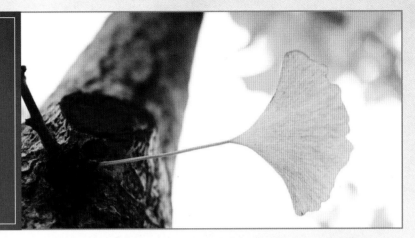

Take 2 to 6 capsules a day (follow package directions) or up to 1 teaspoon (4 droppers full) of tincture a day. The most active ingredients are found in the leaves after they have turned color in the fall.

Cultivation: Ginkgo requires well-drained soil. The trees are largely resistant to insects, drought, and diseases

Propagation: Plant saplings in spring.

Uses: Ginkgo is one of the oldest species of tree on earth. It is used to treat conditions associated with aging, including stroke, heart disease, impotence, deafness, ringing in the ears, blindness, and memory loss. In many studies, it helped people improve their concentration and memory. Ginkgo promotes the action of certain neurotransmitters, chemical compounds responsible for relaying nerve impulses in the brain. It is even undergoing investigation as a treatment for some mental disorders.

Ginkgo increases circulation, including blood flow to the brain, which may help improve memory. Several studies show it reduces the risk of heart attack and improves pain from blood clots (phlebitis) in the legs. Additional studies show that, in a large percentage of people, ginkgo helps impotence caused by narrowing of arteries that supply blood to the penis; macular degeneration of the eyes, a deterioration in vision that may be caused by narrowing of the blood vessels to the eye; and cochlear deafness, which is caused by decreased blood flow to the nerves involved in hearing.

Constituents in ginkgo are potent antioxidants with anti-inflammatory effects. A current scientific theory attributes many of the signs of aging and chronic disease to oxidation of cell membranes by substances called free radicals, which may arise from pollutants or from normal internal production of metabolic substances. Ginkgo counters destruction of cells due to oxidation. Scientists are also investigating ginkgo as a medicine that one day may help the body accept transplanted organs. Researchers also found it can help children with asthma.

The herb produces chemicals that interfere with a substance called platelet activation factor, PAF, which is involved in organ graft rejection, asthma attacks, and blood clots that lead to heart attacks and some strokes.

Part used: Leaves

Preservation: Gather leaves in summer; dry or tincture.

Precautions: Ginkgo may cause problems for people with clotting disorders or those who take blood-thinning medications. Extremely large quantities of ginkgo sometimes cause irritability, restlessness, diarrhea, nausea, and vomiting.

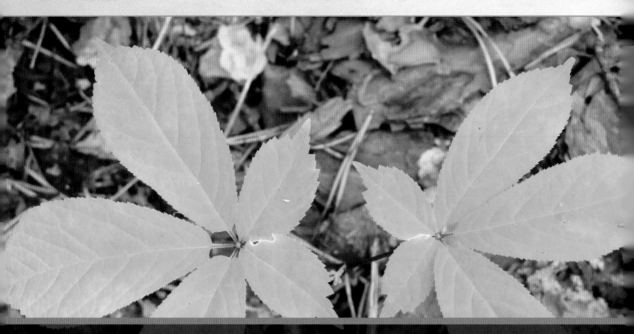

Ginseng, American

Perennial

Botanical Name: *Panax quinquefolius*

Family: Araliaceae

Height: 1 1/2 ft.

Spread: To 1 ft.

Description: American ginseng produces a single stem, a whorl of leaves, and several green-white flowers from June through August. Leaves are toothed; the berries, bright red. American ginseng is indigenous to Manitoba and Quebec and ranges south to Georgia and west through Alabama to Oklahoma. It may be found in hardwood forests on north or northwestern slopes, although years of high demand have made it scarce in the wild.

Ease of care: Difficult

Cultivation: Ginseng needs to be pampered but can be grown in home gardens. The herb demands shade and humusy, rich, well-drained loam. Commercially, ginseng is grown in shelters that mimic forests. The plant must be mulched in winter and takes from five to seven years to produce usable roots, which often fall prey to rotting diseases or gophers.

Propagation: Ginseng seeds require a cold period of at least four months to germinate. The most common way to grow it is to buy seedlings two to three years old.

Uses: The Chinese have used a close relative of American ginseng since prehistoric times. In the United States, colonists grew rich collecting American ginseng and exporting it to China, where the herb enjoys a strong reputation as an aphrodisiac and prolonger of life. Ginseng is an adaptogen, capable of protecting the body from physical and mental stress and helping bodily functions return to normal.

Clinical studies indicate that ginseng may slow the effects of aging, protect cells from free radical damage, prevent heart disease, and help treat anemia, atherosclerosis, depression, diabetes, edema (excess fluid buildup), ulcers, and hypertension. Its complex saponins, ginsenosides, are responsible for most of its actions. They stimulate bone marrow production and immune-system functions, inhibit tumor growth, and detoxify the liver. Ginseng has many dual roles, for example, raising or lowering blood pressure or blood sugar, according to the body's needs.

Ginseng gently stimulates and strengthens the central nervous system, making it useful for treating fatigue and weakness caused by disease and injury. It reduces mental confusion and headaches.

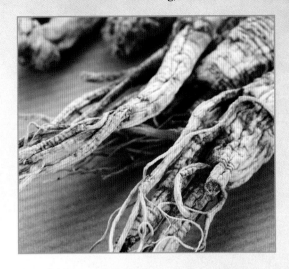

Take about 1 gram of dried root per day. This amount is equivalent to about 4 capsules or 1 to 2 teaspoons tincture (4 to 8 droppers full). Or chew on the whole root. It is also available in a thick concentrated extract to make instant tea and as a sweetened liquid extract. Some herbalists recommend that you take ginseng for several weeks, then stop using it for a week or two for optimum effects.

Part used: Root

Preservation: Do not uproot this endangered plant if you're lucky enough to find it growing wild. Purchase products made from cultivated ginseng, or grow your ginseng. Dry the roots or preserve them in alcohol or honey.

Precautions: Ginseng is generally considered safe. Side effects of taking quantities of ginseng or mixing it with large amounts of caffeine may include some of the symptoms for which it is prescribed, including insomnia, nervousness, and irritability. Consult a physician or qualified herbalist before using ginseng if you have high blood pressure or are pregnant. Use of ginseng aggravates some cases of hypertension and improves other cases.

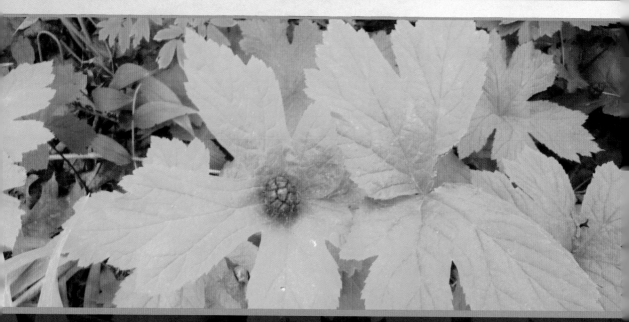

Goldenseal

Perennial

Botanical Name: *Hydrastis canadensis*

Family: Ranunculaceae

Height: 1 ft.

Spread: 1 ft.

Description: Goldenseal is small and erect, with hairy stems growing from a twisted, knotted rhizome that is brown on the outside and bright yellow on the inside. The herb's solitary flowers are white and appear usually in May or June. One or two maple-leaf- shaped leaves appear at the base of the plant. Berries are orange-red and contain two shiny black seeds. Native to North America, the herb is sometimes found in moist, rich woodlands, damp meadows, and forest highlands. Goldenseal is farmed in woodland settings.

Ease of care: Difficult

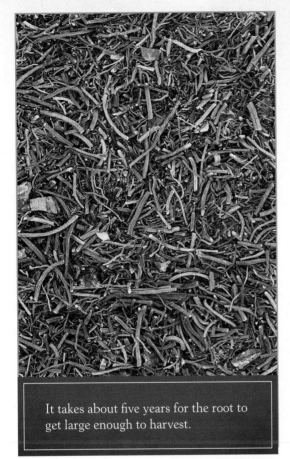

It takes about five years for the root to get large enough to harvest.

depressed appetite, constipation, and urinary and uterine problems.

One of goldenseal's active ingredients is hydrastine, which affects circulation, muscle tone, and uterine contractions. The herb is also an antiseptic, astringent, and antibiotic, making it effective for treating eye and other types of infections. Berberine and related alkaloids have been credited with goldenseal's antimicrobial effects. Goldenseal makes a good antiseptic skin wash for wounds and for internal skin surfaces, such as in the vagina and ear; it also treats canker sores and infected gums. The herb has been found to fight a number of disease-causing microbes, including *Staphylococcus* and *Streptococcus* organisms.

Berberine may be responsible for increasing white blood cell activity and promoting blood flow in the liver and spleen. Berberine has been used in China to combat the reduction of white blood cells that commonly follows chemotherapy and radiation treatment for cancer. Studies suggest it may have potential in the treatment of brain and skin cancers.

You can drink up to 2 cups a day of tea, but the taste is very bitter. Take 1/2 to 1 teaspoon tincture (2 to 4 droppers full) up to twice a day or dab on minor cuts or sore, inflamed gums.

Cultivation: Overharvesting of wild plants has put goldenseal on the endangered list. (You can use Oregon grape root as an alternative to goldenseal. It also contains goldenseal's active ingredient, berberine, and is much less expensive).

Propagation: Sow seeds in fall or stratify them. New plants also grow from root division.

Uses: The Cherokee Indians mixed powdered goldenseal root with bear grease and slathered their bodies to protect themselves from mosquitoes and other insects. Pioneers adopted the herb and used it to treat wounds, rashes, mouth sores, morning sickness, liver and stomach complaints, internal hemorrhaging,

Part used: Root

Preservation: Harvest roots in late fall and dry slowly.

Precautions: Hydrastine accumulates in the system and is toxic in large doses. Berberine may lower blood pressure, but hydrastine raises it, so avoid the herb if you have high blood pressure, heart disease, or glaucoma, except under professional guidance.

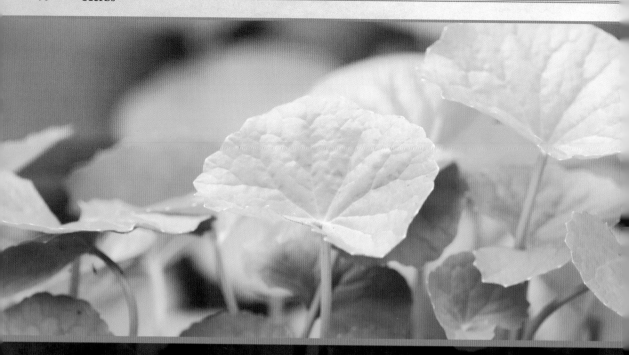

Gotu Kola

Perennial

Botanical Name: *Centella asiatica*

Family: Apiaceae (Umbelliferae)

Height: 6 in.

Spread: 6 in.; may become invasive

Description: Gotu kola is a plant of many names. It produces fan-shaped leaves about the size of an old British penny; hence, its names include Indian pennywort, marsh penny, and water pennywort. Gotu kola is related to carrot, parsley, dill, and fennel but has neither the feathery leaves of its cousins nor the umbrella of tiny flowers they produce.

Ease of care: Moderate

Cultivation: Gotu kola grows wild in marshy areas. Although it is a perennial, it grows only as an annual in cool climates. The plant requires moist, rich soil and partial shade. To thrive, gotu kola needs humidity, thus, it's best suited for subtropical climates or a greenhouse.

Propagation: Seeds germinate in seven to ten days. The plant may be propagated by means of layering.

Uses: Gotu kola is considered a relaxant, nerve tonic, diuretic, anti-inflammatory, and wound healer. The herb has long been regarded as a life extender. Shepherds in Sri Lanka noticed that elephants ate it and lived a long time. Thus, a later proverb reasoned, "Two leaves a day will keep old age away." Indian Ayurvedic physicians have used the plant extensively to treat the problems of aging. There is no evidence to support the theory that gotu kola prolongs life, but some tests have shown that the plant is a sedative and tonic for the nervous system and could help in treating many neurologic and mental disturbances, especially debility stemming from stress. Ayurvedics also use gotu kola to treat asthma, anemia, and other blood disorders.

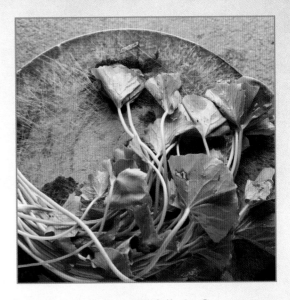

In India gotu kola has been called brahmi, in honor of the god Brahma. It is reputed to improve memory, and East Indians again note that elephants, which supposedly never forget, consider gotu kola a delicacy.

The plant also has been used internally to treat rheumatism and other inflammatory ailments. In many Asian countries, physicians employ gotu kola leaves and roots to treat wounds, ulcers, and lesions that don't heal properly, including leprosy lesions. Gotu kola contains a chemical called asiaticoside, which aids in the treatment of leprosy. It also helps prevent scarring, and it has been used successfully in Germany to heal the skin after surgery.

Gotu kola is thought to stimulate the body's immune system. It improves circulation throughout the body—one reason it may improve memory and brain function. It also improves varicose veins and other circulation disorders.

Part used: Leaves, stems

Preservation: Use fresh leaves anytime. Leaves may also be dried and infused for creams, lotions, and ointments.

Precautions: In moderate doses, gotu kola is considered quite safe. Although mice developed tumors after the concentrated chemical asiaticoside was applied to their skin, newer evidence demonstrated that a gotu kola tincture inhibits the growth of cancer cells in smaller doses. Don't take gotu kola if you are pregnant or nursing or if you take tranquilizers because gotu kola's sedating properties may interfere with the drug. In extremely large doses, gotu kola is narcotic, producing rashes or dizziness. If you develop these symptoms, stop using the herb.

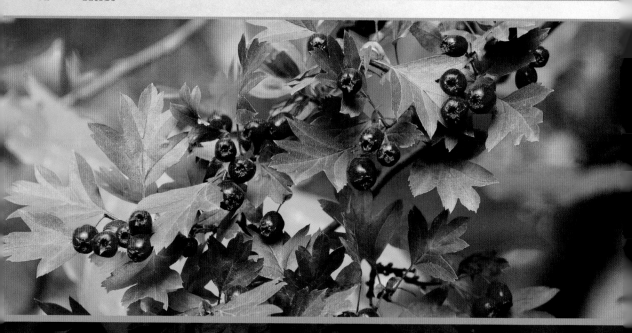

Hawthorn

Perennial

Botanical Name: *Crataegus laevigata*

Family: Rosaceae

Height: To 25 ft.

Spread: To 10 ft.

Description: Like many members of the rose family, hawthorn bears thorns as well as lovely, fragrant flowers and brightly pigmented berries high in vitamin C. As many as 900 species of hawthorn exist in North America, ranging from deciduous trees to thorny-branched shrubs. Hawthorn produces white flower clusters in May. The herb is native to Europe, with closely related species in North Africa and western Asia. It is often found in areas with hedges and deciduous woods.

Ease of care: Easy

Cultivation: Hawthorn tolerates a wide variety of soils but prefers ground that is alkaline, rich, loamy, and moist. Hawthorn also likes full sun. The tree sometimes falls prey to aphids and other insects and fungus.

Propagation: Sow seed in the spring. Certain varieties of hawthorn must be grafted or budded. Smaller trees transplant better than larger ones. Trees are sold in most nurseries.

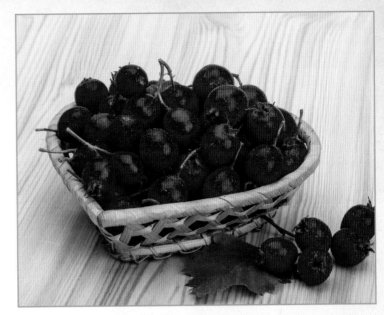

Uses: Hawthorn has been cherished for centuries. The Druids considered hawthorn a sacred tree. The Pilgrims brought it to America: Mayflower is, in fact, another name for hawthorn.

Hawthorn is an important herb for treating heart conditions. The berries and flowers contain several complex chemical constituents, including flavonoids such as anthocyanidins, which improve the strength of capillaries and reduce damage to blood vessels from oxidizing agents. Hawthorn's ability to dilate blood vessels, enhancing circulation, makes it useful for treating angina, atherosclerosis, high and low blood pressure, and elevated cholesterol levels. Many clinical studies have demonstrated its effectiveness for such conditions—with the use of hawthorn, the heart requires less oxygen when under stress. Heart action is normalized and becomes stronger and more efficient. Hawthorn also helps balance the heart's rhythm and is prescribed for arrhythmias and heart palpitations by European physicians. Although it affects the heart somewhat like the medication digitalis, hawthorn does not have a cumulative effect on the heart.

Take 1/2 to 1 teaspoon tincture (2 to 4 droppers full) up to five times a day, or drink up to 5 cups of the tea. It is often combined with other heart tonics such as motherwort and garlic.

Part used: Berries, twigs behind the flowers, and flowers

Preservation: Gather flowers in spring and tincture. Gather berries in fall and dry or tincture. You can also use berries to make jam or jelly.

Precautions: Hawthorn is considered safe and may be used for long periods. Do not self-medicate with hawthorn. Consult a physician or herbalist before taking it, especially if you take prescription heart medication: Hawthorn may intensify the effects of these drugs.

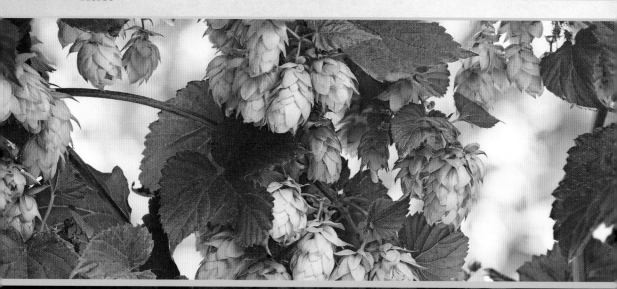

Hops

Perennial

Botanical Name: *Humulus lupulus*

Family: Cannabaceae

Height: 20–40 ft.

Spread: Spreading vine

Description: Like the grape, hops is a quick-growing and quick-spreading vine. Each year a stem grows from the root and begins to twine. After the third year, hops produces a papery, conelike fruit called a strobile. Male and female flowers grow on separate plants and appear from middle to late summer. Hops leaves somewhat resemble grape leaves, hairy and coarse, with serrated edges. A relative of marijuana, hops is native to Europe and can be found in vacant fields and along rivers. The Pilgrims brought hops to Massachusetts, and it quickly spread south to Virginia. Most hops grown in the United States is for the beer industry, which uses hops to flavor its products.

Ease of care: Easy

Cultivation: Hops can be grown as a garden plant. Vines also are grown commercially in hopyards on wires strung between poles. Hops requires full sun, deep, humusy, well-drained soil, and good air circulation to prevent mildew from forming.

Propagation: Hops may be started from cuttings or suckers taken in early summer from healthy old plants.

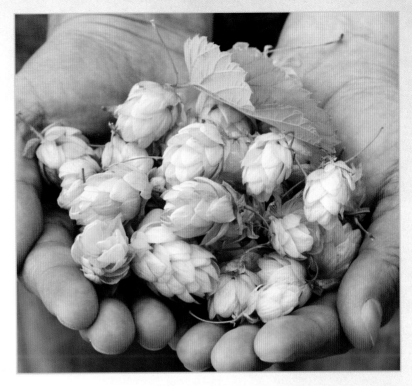

Uses: If you worked in a hopyard, you might find yourself falling asleep on the job. Hops contains chemicals that depress the central nervous system, making it a useful sedative herb. Both Abraham Lincoln and England's King George III, notorious insomniacs, reportedly lay their heads on hops-filled pillows to ensure a good night's sleep. Hops' other constituents are antiseptic, antibacterial, and anti-inflammatory, and they slightly increase activity of the female hormone estrogen. Hops has also been used as a pain reliever, fever cure, expectorant, and diuretic. It has been prescribed to treat nervous heart conditions, PMS, menstrual pain, and nervous symptoms of menopause. The Greeks and Romans used hops as a digestive aid. If you have drunk beer, you will be familiar with hops' pleasantly bitter taste. This bitterness also makes hops an excellent digestive aid. Since the 9th century AD, brewers have used hops to flavor and preserve beer. In some Scandinavian coun-tries, weavers make a coarse cloth from hops vine. Dried hops also makes an interesting addition to dried floral arrangements.

Drink hops tea up to three times a day. Take 1/2 to 1 teaspoon (2 to 4 droppers full) of tincture up to three times a day or take it in pills. Hops is often mixed with other sedative herbs or herbs that help relieve menstrual or menopausal symptoms.

Part used: Fruit

Preservation: Gather strobiles in summer after they turn an amber color; dry or tincture. Tincturing is the best way to preserve hops. The herb becomes unstable in the presence of light and air and loses some of its flavor and medicinal effectiveness.

Precautions: The herb may cause a rash known as hops dermatitis. Avoid hops if you're pregnant because of its hormonal actions.

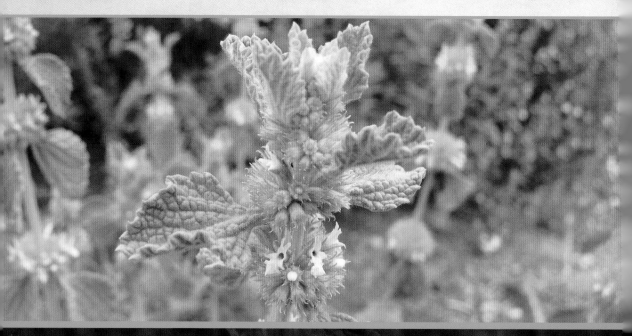

Horehound

Perennial

Botanical Name: *Marrubium vulgare*

Family: Lamiaceae (Labiatae)

Height: 1–2 ft.

Spread: 8–12 in.

Description: A member of the mint family, horehound has branching stems, which may give it a bushy appearance. Leaves have a "woolly" look, and flowers appear in dense white whorls in summer. Horehound is native to southern Europe, central and western Asia, and North Africa. It has become naturalized throughout North America. You'll find it in sandy wastelands, pastures, vacant lots, and abandoned fields.

Ease of care: Easy

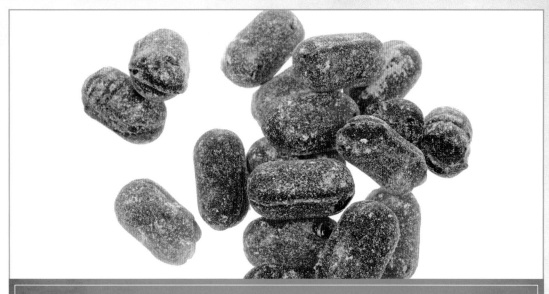

Today some people use the leaves to make an old-fashioned candy called horehound drops.

Cultivation: Horehound is a hardy plant in zone 4 that prefers deep, well-drained, sandy soil and full sun. It may become invasive.

Propagation: Horehound grows easily from seed or division in spring.

Uses: When your grandfather had a cold, he may have sucked on a horehound lozenge. The herb has been used for centuries to open clogged nasal passages and alleviate other symptoms associated with the sniffles. One of the Hebrew's ritual bitter herbs, horehound was also prized by the Greeks and Egyptians. Herbalists have employed it to treat hepatitis and jaundice. But horehound's most reliable uses are to soothe sore throats, help the lungs expel mucus, and treat bronchitis. A weak sedative, it also helps normalize an irregular heartbeat. It induces sweating and will lower a fever, especially when infused and drunk as a hot tea.

The herb's primary constituents include an essential oil, tannin, and a bitter chemical called marrubiin. The plant also contains vitamin C, which adds to its ability to fight colds. Horehound has a taste similar to sage and hyssop but more bitter. At one time it was used in England as a bitter to flavor ale.

If you can handle the bitter taste, drink horehound tea, but more likely you'll use it as a tincture or cough syrup. Take 1/4 to 1/2 teaspoon (1 to 2 droppers full) of tincture up to three times a day. Take the syrup a teaspoon at a time. Horehound preparations typically include other herbs used for lung congestion such as mullein or elecampane. The lozenges often contain anise to improve their taste.

Part used: Leaves

Preservation: Gather leaves before the herb blooms in summer; dry or tincture.

Precautions: In very large doses, horehound may cause cardiac arrhythmias.

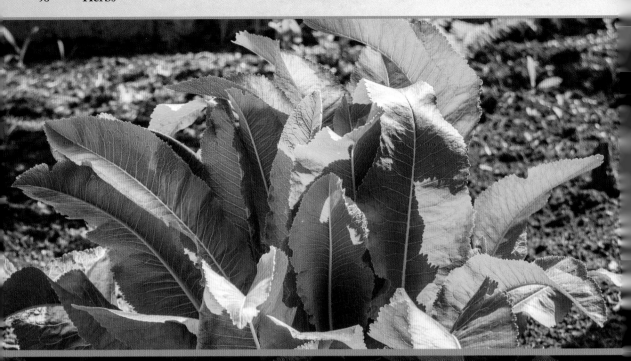

Horseradish

Perennial

Botanical Name: *Armoracia rusticana*

Family: Cruciferae

Height: 4–5 ft.

Spread: 2 ft.

Description: Horseradish, a cousin of mustard, produces a long tapering root. Its flowers are small and white and appear in midsummer; its leaves are abundant. Native to southeastern Europe and western Asia, the herb is cultivated widely in North America and naturalized in some areas.

Ease of care: Easy

Cultivation: Horseradish prefers average, moist, heavy soil and full sun. Once established, it is difficult to eradicate. Some gardeners believe that planting horseradish near potatoes makes them more disease-resistant.

Propagation: Take cuttings 8 to 9 inches long from the root in the spring. Each cutting should have a bud. Place them 12 inches apart in soil that is at least 12 to 15 inches deep.

Uses: Have you ever bitten into a roast beef sandwich and thought your nose was on fire? The sandwich probably contained horseradish. Even a tiny taste of this potent condiment seems to go straight to your nose. Whether it's on a roast beef sandwich or in an herbal preparation, horseradish clears sinuses, increases circulation, and promotes expulsion of mucus from upper respiratory passages.

Horseradish has been used as a medicine for centuries. Its chief constituent decomposes upon exposure to air to turn into mustard oil, which gives both horseradish and mustard their heat and flavor. The root contains an antibiotic substance and vitamin C, which are effective in clearing up sinus, bronchial, and urinary infections. Horseradish can make an effective heat-producing poultice that alleviates the pain of arthritis and neuralgia. It also stimulates digestion and has long been eaten with fatty foods to help digest them.

As a condiment, horseradish is widely used. Its sharp mustardy taste enhances mayonnaise, fish, beef, sausage, eggs, potatoes, and beets. Horseradish is used extensively in Eastern European cuisine and is a featured ingredient in Dresden sauce. Tender new leaves may be chopped fine and tossed in salads.

Grate the fresh root in a food processor or blender. Add vinegar and honey or sugar to taste. Spread 1/4 teaspoon or less of prepared horseradish on a cracker and eat it. Stir horseradish in a sip of warm water with a little honey and take for hoarseness or head congestion, or take 1/2 teaspoon tincture (2 droppers full) in warm water. Repeat every hour until the problem clears.

Part used: Root. Fresh root is superior as both medicine and food, but dried horseradish powder will do in a pinch.

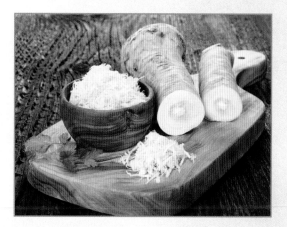

Preservation: Harvest roots in late fall. Store whole in dry sand in a cool, dark place. Horseradish roots will stay fresh for months. The best way to preserve horseradish is to put it in vinegar or lemon juice right after grating it; the mustard oil produced upon grating is quickly lost otherwise. Use grated horseradish within three months. Reconstitute dried horseradish at least 30 minutes before serving.

Precautions: Large doses of horseradish may cause an upset stomach, vomiting, or headache. Topical use may cause inflammation. Horseradish's volatile fumes may irritate the lungs if you inhale large quantities on a continuous basis.

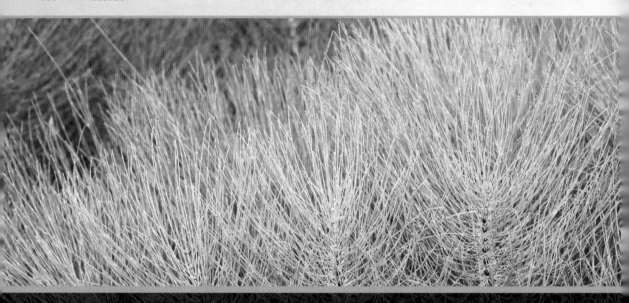

Horsetail

Perennial

Botanical Name: *Equisetum arvense*

Family: Equisetaceae

Height: 1st stage, 4–8 in.; 2nd stage, to 1 1/2 ft.

Spread: 6 in.

Description: One of the planet's oldest plant species, horsetail has been around for 200 million years. The herb's name refers to the resemblance of the whorls of its needlelike leaves to a horse's tail. The herb's other common name, scouring rush, derives from the plant's one-time use as a natural scouring pad for pots and pans. Horsetail appears in two stages: In the first, the herb produces a green-yellowish bamboolike stalk; in the second, whorls of threadlike leaves appear around the stalk. Harvest it in this second stage in the spring while it is still young. You're likely to encounter this hardy herb in moist woods, along roads, and in waste places.

Ease of care: Easy

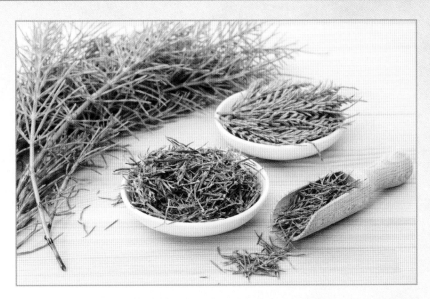

Cultivation: Horsetail prefers acidic to neutral, humusy, moist soil and partial shade. You can purchase horsetail at many nurseries. Once it has rooted, it's difficult to eradicate. Try planting the herb in a bucket placed just below the surface of a pond.

Propagation: Horsetails are easy to divide. Dig and divide the roots.

Uses: Horsetail is high in minerals, particularly silica. The herb contains so much silica, in fact, that you can use it to polish metal. Early Americans used horsetail to scour pots and pans. Horsetail treats water retention, bed-wetting, and other bladder problems, including kidney stones. It is also used to decrease an enlarged prostate. Used externally, it stops bleeding and helps wounds to heal. It was once used to prevent the lungs from scarring in people with tuberculosis.

Because it contains minerals, horsetail strengthens bone, hair, and fingernails. Horsetail infusions—often combined with nettles—are drunk to help broken bones mend. The silica in it encourages the absorption of calcium by the body and helps prevent build-up of fatty deposits in the arteries.

Drink up to 2 cups a day of the tea. Take 1/2 to 1 teaspoon tincture (2 to 4 droppers full) or 2 capsules up to two times a day. You can buy capsules of horsetail mixed with other herbs and nutrients to strengthen nails and hair. It's best to take horsetail for a week and abstain for two before resuming use. It is usually blended with other herbs such as saw palmetto and nettle root to treat an enlarged prostate.

Dried stems are interesting additions to flower arrangements. Horsetail yields a yellowish-green dye.

Part used: Stems, shoots

Preservation: Gather very young shoots in spring and cook as you would asparagus. Horsetail branches are also made into infusions and tinctures.

Precautions: Make sure your horsetail was not gathered near an industrial site. Horsetail tends to pick up large amounts of nitrates and selenium from the soil. Equisetene, a chemical found in the plant, is a nerve toxin in large doses. It increases in amount as the plant matures, so pick horsetail only in the spring when it is in its second stage. Long-term use of horsetail could result in kidney damage. Do not use horsetail if you have high blood pressure or are pregnant.

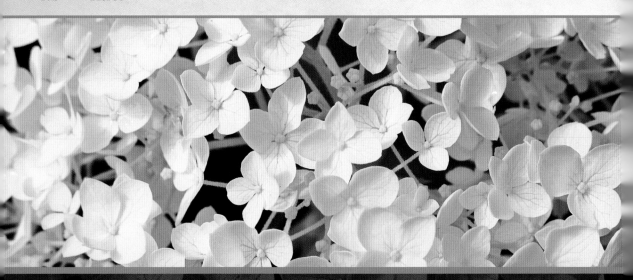

Hydrangea

Perennial

Botanical Name: *Hydrangea arborescens*

Family: Saxifragaceae

Height: To 9 ft.

Spread: To 6 ft.

Description: Native to North America, hydrangea is also known as seven barks because it produces seven separate layers of different-colored bark. In the wild, 23 species are related to this well-known cultivated plant. Many cousins are found in eastern Asia and the Americas. Hydrangea flowers are pink to deep blue, depending on soil alkalinity levels. The plant flowers from July through September, sometimes later. Leaves are ovate (egg-shaped), toothed, and pointed. In the wild, hydrangea is found in rich woods from New York to Florida and west from Louisiana to Ohio. The plant is highly regarded for its garden beauty.

Ease of care: Easy

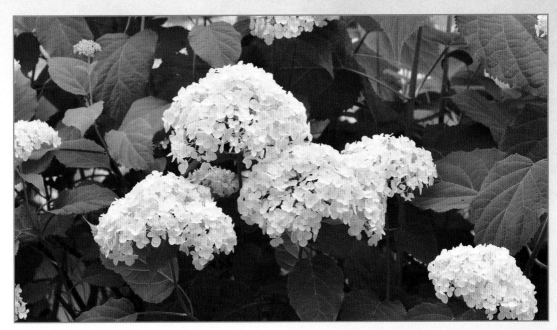

Cultivation: Hydrangea prefers rich, moist soil and full sun or partial shade.

Propagation: Cuttings, layering

Uses: Hydrangea root, which contains a number of glycosides, saponins, and resins, is used most often for treating enlarged prostate glands. The herb is employed to treat urinary stones and cystitis, and it can help prevent the recurrence of kidney stones. But you should not self-medicate for urinary or kidney stones, as these conditions require professional medical treatment.

The root is a laxative and diuretic. American Indians used its bark in poultices for treating wounds, burns, sore muscles, sprains, and tumors, and they chewed it for stomach and heart trouble. The leaves also contain some of the medicine but are not as strong as the roots. You can dry the flower heads as well as the individual flowers for use in craft projects. To retain their color, dry them as quickly as possible in a dark place or dry them in silica gel. The flowers are also very attractive when pressed.

Drink 1 cup of tea, three times a day. If using tincture, take 1/2 to 3/4 teaspoon (2 to 3 droppers full), three times a day. To prevent kidney stones, hydrangea is generally mixed with other herbs such as horsetail, Joe-pye weed, goldenrod, cramp bark, and dandelion. You may also find it combined with saw palmetto, nettle root, horsetail, marshmallow, and other herbs that reduce prostate inflammation.

Part used: Dried roots and rhizome; flowers for dried flower projects

Preservation: Harvest roots in autumn; clean and slice while fresh because the roots become very hard after they dry. Pick the flowers just before they are in full bloom.

Precautions: Hydrangea may cause dizziness and indigestion when ingested in large amounts. Lower the dose if this occurs. The wood is reported to cause skin reactions in woodworkers, and the flowers have been known to make children sick when they ate the buds.

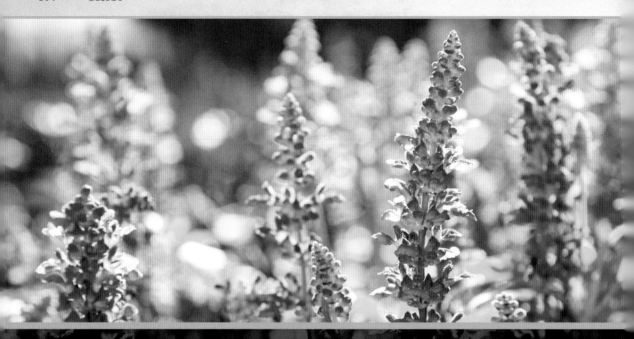

Hyssop

Perennial

Botanical Name: *Hyssopus officinalis*

Family: Lamiaceae (Labiatae)

Height: 1 1/2–2 ft.

Spread: 1 ft.

Description: Hyssop is a compact, aromatic member of the mint family, with many branches and square stems. Its leaves have a minty, somewhat medicinal odor. Blue or violet flowers appear in whorls to form dense spikes at the top of the stem from June through August. Hyssop is native to the Mediterranean and has become naturalized in some areas of North America.

Ease of care: Easy

Cultivation: Hyssop prefers light, well-drained soil and full sun. Aside from occasional pruning, the plant requires little care.

Propagation: Sow seeds in the spring; take cuttings or divide in the spring or fall.

Uses: Hyssop has been a favorite medicinal herb since it was used in ancient Greece. With its strong camphor-like odor, the herb was strewn on floors to freshen homes in the Middle Ages. Hyssop baths were once used in England to treat rheumatism. Hyssop, which has a chemistry similar to horehound, has been used mostly to treat bronchitis, flu, colds, and sore throats. It reduces inflammation, so it makes a good throat gargle. In laboratory tests, it destroys the herpesvirus. A poultice of the fresh leaves promotes healing of wounds. The herb's essential oil is a prime flavoring of liqueurs, including Benedictine and Chartreuse. Add leaves to salads, chicken soup, fruit dishes, lamb, and poultry stuffing. Hyssop essential oil is expensive and found in quality perfumes. Use the herb or essential oil in a cleansing facial steam. Hyssop is said to repel flea beetles and other pests.

Hyssop is rarely used in tinctures; instead it is added to teas and syrups to treat congestion, colds, and flu. Drink up to 2 cups of tea or take 2 tablespoons of syrup daily.

Part used: Leaves

Preservation: Harvest stems just before flowers open. Hang in a warm, dry place. Harvest flowers as soon as they bloom, and dry or tincture. Harvest only green matter; hyssop's tough woody stems have less oil than the leaves do. Store dried hyssop in tightly covered glass containers or tins.

Precautions: Use hyssop in small doses and not at all if you are pregnant or have high blood pressure. It can also induce epileptic seizures. Be especially cautious when using the essential oil, which is more potent than the plant.

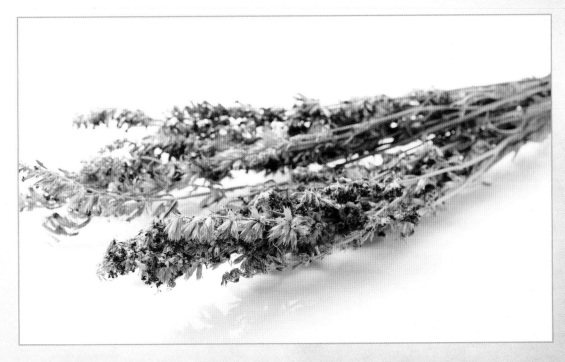

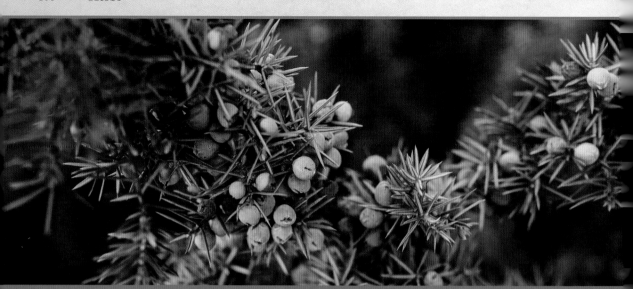

Juniper

Perennial

Botanical Name: *Juniperus communis*

Family: Cupressaceae

Height: 2–20 ft.

Spread: From 4 ft.

Description: Most junipers are low growing, with tangled, spreading branches covered with reddish-brown bark. The many varieties of juniper vary in size, color, and shape. Most cultivated junipers are dwarf varieties. The tree produces male and female flowers on separate plants. Juniper blooms from April through June and produces berries that ripen to a bluish-purple in the tree's second year. The berries are covered with a whitish wax, and its leaves are green, prickly, and needle-shaped. This species is native to Europe and has become naturalized throughout North America.

Ease of care: Easy

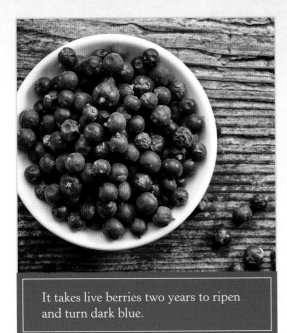

It takes live berries two years to ripen and turn dark blue.

Cultivation: Hardy trees, junipers will grow just about anywhere. They prefer full sun and sandy or light, loamy soil. To produce berries, you must grow both male and female plants. Once established, junipers require little care.

Propagation: Sow seed in the spring or fall, but germination may take two to three years. In late summer, take cuttings, which root easily if kept moist. Seedlings, available at nurseries, may be transplanted at any time of year, although they do better in early spring or fall.

Uses: The berries give gin its distinct flavor. American Indians used the leaves and berries externally to cure infections, relieve arthritis, and treat wounds. Adding a handful of crushed juniper leaves to a warm bath soothes aching muscles. A compress of juniper berries is sometimes recommended for gout, rheumatoid arthritis, and nerve, muscle, joint, and tendon pain. The berries were once chewed by doctors to ward off

infection when treating patients. Chewing them also improves bad breath.

Juniper's essential oils relieve coughs and lung congestion. Its tars and resins treat psoriasis and other skin conditions. In both treatments, juniper has a warming, circulation-stimulating action. Juniper also relieves gas in the digestive system, increases stomach acid, and is a diuretic. The essential oil in its berries has antiseptic properties and is sometimes used for chronic urinary tract infections.

In the kitchen, you can use juniper berries to flavor patés and sauerkraut. Crushed berries spice game dishes, stews, sauces, and marinades. Toss juniper branches on the grill to impart a distinctive smoky taste to meats.

Drink up to 1 cup of tea a day. Take the tea or tincture for one week, then abstain for one or two. Take 10 to 20 drops of tincture no more than four times a day. To make a massage oil, dilute juniper berry essential oil with vegetable oil. Rub on the skin over the urinary tract or digestive tract.

Part used: Berries, leaves

Preservation: Harvest leaves at any time; wear gloves because leaves are prickly. Harvest only ripe berries. Spread berries on a screen and dry until they turn black. Tincture crushed juniper berries or store whole.

Precautions: Don't use juniper if you're pregnant or have a kidney infection or chronic kidney problems. Overdose symptoms may include diarrhea, intestinal pain, kidney pain, blood in urine, rapid heartbeat, and elevated blood pressure. Some hay fever sufferers develop allergic reactions to juniper. Don't use juniper if you develop any reactions. Use the essential oil externally only and with caution since it is very potent.

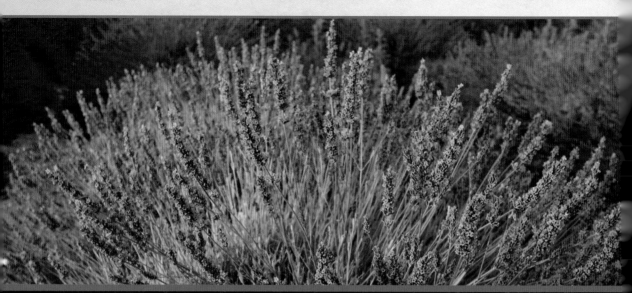

Lavender

Perennial

Botanical Name: *Lavandula angustifolia*

Family: Lamiaceae (Labiatae)

Height: 2–4 ft.

Spread: 2–3 ft.

Description: Lavender is a bushy plant with silver-gray, narrow leaves. It produces abundant 1 1/2–2-foot flower stalks topped by fragrant and attractive purple-blue flower clusters. The plant flowers in June and July. An outstanding addition to any garden design, the herb also makes a nice edging or potted plant. There are a number of species and cultivars of lavender. Differences focus primarily on flower color (some have white, others, pink flowers), size, and growth habits. Munstead, a smaller variety of lavender, may be clipped to form a low hedge. Lavender is native to the Mediterranean, but the herb is cultivated around the world.

Ease of care: Easy

Cultivation: Lavender prefers full sun in well-drained, sandy to poor, alkaline soil.

Propagation: Sow seed in spring; take cuttings or layer before the plant flowers.

Uses: Perhaps the smell of lavender reminds you of soap. That's because lavender is a prime ingredient of many soaps. Its name, in fact, derives from the Latin "to wash." The Romans and Greeks used lavender in the bath. Lavender is also found commercially in shaving creams, colognes, and perfumes. It is used in many cosmetics and aromatherapy products because it is so versatile, and its fragrance blends so well with other herbs. Studies show that the scent is very relaxing. Lavender's scent is also a remedy for headache and nervous tension.

Lavender cosmetics are good for all complexion types. It is an excellent skin healer: It promotes the healing of burns, abrasions, infected sores, and other types of inflammations, including varicose veins. It is also a popular hair rinse. The herb is a carminative (relieves gas and bowel pain) and antispasmodic. It is most often used for sore muscles in the form of a massage oil. As recently as World War I, lavender was used in the field as a disinfectant for wounds; herbalists still recommend it for that purpose. Lavender destroys several viruses, including many that cause colds and flu. It also relieves lung and sinus congestion. Lavender flowers may be added to vinegars, jellies, sachets, and potpourri. Place a sprig of lavender in a drawer to freshen linens. And dried flowers make wonderful herbal arrangements, although they are fragile.

It is rare to find lavender included in herbal teas, tinctures, or pills, but the essential oil is one of the most popular for use in skin care preparations. A few drops can be added to creams, salves, lotions, or the bath. Lavender makes an excellent compress for a headache, sore eyes, or a skin injury. For sinus and lung congestion, use a lavender steam. Add a strong lavender infusion or a couple drops of the essential oil to a quart of warm water for a douche to treat vaginal infections with *Candida* fungus.

Part used: Leaves, flowers, branches

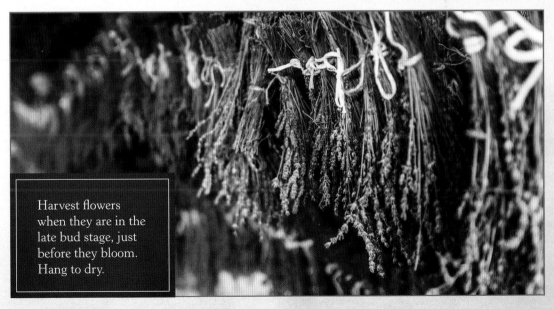

Harvest flowers when they are in the late bud stage, just before they bloom. Hang to dry.

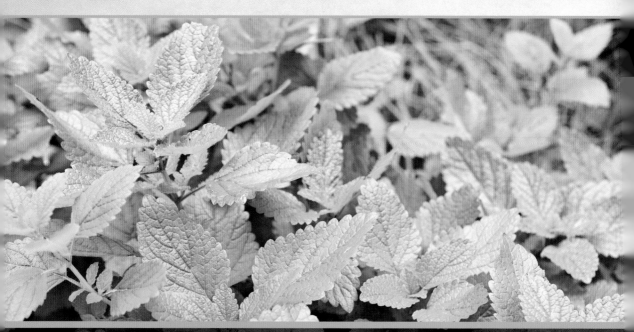

Lemon Balm

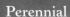

Perennial

Botanical Name: *Melissa officinalis*

Family: Lamiaceae (Labiatae)

Height: 3 ft.

Spread: 1–2 ft.

Description: Lemon balm is an attractive plant with shield-shaped leaves that smell strongly of lemon. Like most mints, the herb produces square stems and flowers from July through September. Lemon balm is native to Europe and North Africa but has become naturalized elsewhere, including many parts of the United States. It is cultivated throughout the world.

Ease of care: Easy

Cultivation: Lemon balm prospers in full sun but will also do well in partial shade. It likes a well-drained or moist, sandy soil. The plant grows abundantly. It attracts honeybees but repels other insects. Lemon balm is susceptible to developing powdery mildew, so avoid overhead watering if this is a problem. It is susceptible to frost and may need to be mulched during the winter in a cold climate.

Propagation: Sow seeds or divide in autumn or early spring; take cuttings in spring and summer. However, lemon balm self-seeds so profusely, you may need only to transplant it once after it is established.

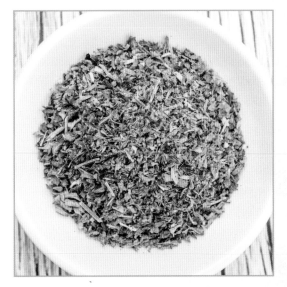

Uses: This venerable herb has been used for at least 2,000 years. Homer mentions the balm in his epic *Odyssey*. And Greek and Roman physicians prescribed it to treat injuries from scorpions and dogs. But lemon balm's real fans were the Arabs, who believed it was good for disorders of the heart and dispelling melancholy. Colonists brought lemon balm to America. Thomas Jefferson grew it at Monticello, and many Old Williamsburg recipes call for its use.

Lemon balm was an important medicine well into the 19th century. The herb acts as a mild tranquilizer and is used to soothe a nervous stomach or minor heart palpitations. Its calming effect combined with its antihistamine action make it an excellent choice for relieving mild headaches; it's especially useful for children.

Researchers have found that a mixture of lemon balm and valerian is as effective as some tranquilizers, without the side effects. The scent alone has long been used to reduce nervous tension. Compounds in it may even prove useful to people with hyperthyroidism, although the herb itself won't replace thyroid medication. And its essential oil reduces risk of infections by inhibiting growth of bacteria and viruses. Recent studies show it is particularly effective against the herpesvirus. It is also effective against flu and colds.

In the kitchen, this herb, with its lemony-mint flavor, complements salads, fruits, marinated vegetables, poultry and stuffing, punch, fish marinades, and an assortment of vegetables, including corn, broccoli, asparagus, and beans. Lemon balm is employed commercially to flavor liqueurs such as Benedictine and Chartreuse. Lemon balm infusions cleanse the skin and help clear up acne. You may add leaves to your bath—or even polish furniture with them.

You can enjoy lemon balm tea freely. It is delicious hot or iced, by itself or mixed with other herbs. It is often blended with chamomile and mint as a digestive aid, for relaxation, or to give to children as a calmative.

Part used: Leaves

Preservation: Harvest in midsummer and hang branches to dry, or spread leaves on screens.

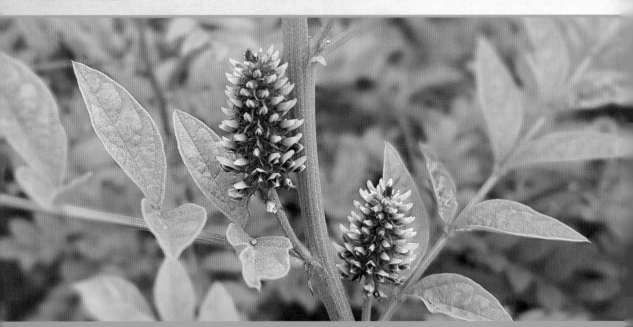

Licorice

Perennial

Botanical Name: *Glycyrrhiza glabra*

Family: Fabaceae (Leguminosae)

Height: To 3 ft.

Spread: 2 ft.

Description: Licorice sends out stolons that create a tangled mass of taproots. The herb flowers in midsummer; in climates with a long growing season, the herb produces a fruit pod clustered in a prickly pod. Licorice is native to the Mediterranean region, northern India, and southwest Asia. It is cultivated in Greece, Iran, Iraq, India, Spain, Syria, and Russia.

Ease of care: Moderate

Cultivation: Licorice prefers neutral, well-drained, sandy soil and full sun to partial shade. In cold climates, take the plants inside during the winter. Licorice will handle only a light frost.

Propagation: Sow seed in early spring or late fall; take cuttings from suckers.

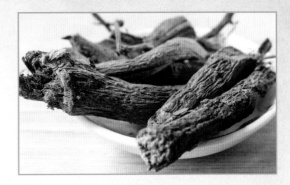

Uses: Licorice has been a popular flavoring for millennia. Archaeologists have determined that the Assyrians and Egyptians used it. Licorice's main constituent, glycyrrhizin, is 50 times sweeter than sugar. Although the herb was once a popular candy flavoring, most of the licorice candy made in the United States is actually flavored with anise. Licorice is used commercially in pastries, ice cream, puddings, soy sauce, soy-based meat substitutes, and tobacco.

As a medicine, licorice was also used by the Greeks and Romans and is still one of the most popular Chinese herbs. In the United States, licorice is in cough syrups and drops. The herb is also used to sweeten mouthwash and toothpaste. A laxative, this soothing herb has also been prescribed for stomach and bowel inflammation and peptic ulcers. Licorice reduces stomach acid and encourages the stomach to protect itself from acid. Carbenoxolene, a compound derived from licorice, was, until recently, the drug of choice to treat ulcers. Another form of licorice, deglycyrrhizinated licorice, shows promise as a future drug. Studies show it can be as effective as Tagemet and Zantac. Licorice has estrogenic effects and is useful for treating menopausal symptoms and normalizing an irregular menstrual cycle. Licorice is also an antiviral and decongestant and is used to treat dermatitis, colds, and infections. It enhances the immune system, and it may have anti-tumor properties. Several clinical studies indicate it may be useful to treat herpes, a viral condition which currently has no cure.

Like the adrenal hormone cortisone, it decreases inflammation, so it is used to reduce the symptoms of rheumatoid arthritis and other inflammatory disorders but without cortisone's side effects. And while cortisone therapy depletes the adrenal glands, licorice encourages them to function better and relieves adrenal exhaustion. Studies show licorice neutralizes liver toxins and increases the liver's ability to store glycogen, which provides muscles with energy.

Take licorice in the form of syrup, tea, tincture, or pills. Use no more than 1 cup of tea or 1/8 teaspoon (1/2 dropper full) of tincture a day. You can also chew on the dried roots.

Part used: Root

Preservation: Dig roots in late autumn or early winter. Leave sections of the root in the soil to sprout the next year. Dry licorice in shade.

Precautions: Licorice may raise blood pressure in people who have hypertension. It may cause headaches, shortness of breath, bloating, and fluid retention in high doses or with long-term use of low daily doses. Avoid licorice if you're pregnant. Do not use as a daily laxative as it can cause excessive potassium loss.

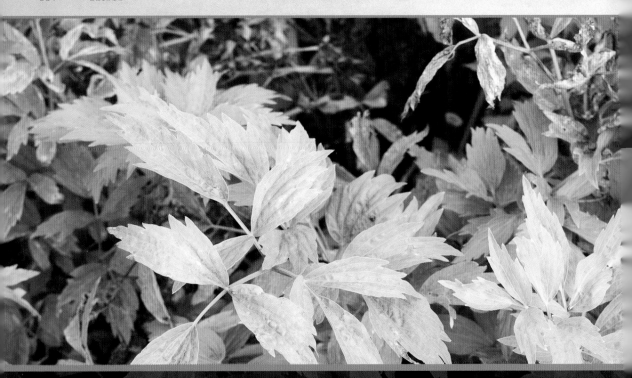

Lovage

Perennial

Botanical Name: *Levisticum officinalis*

Family: Apiaceae (Umbelliferae)

Height: 4–6 ft.

Spread: 2 ft., spreads

Description: A large plant, lovage produces glossy, dark green leaves that resemble those of celery. The herb flowers in June and July. It is native to southern Europe and has become naturalized throughout North America.

Ease of care: Easy

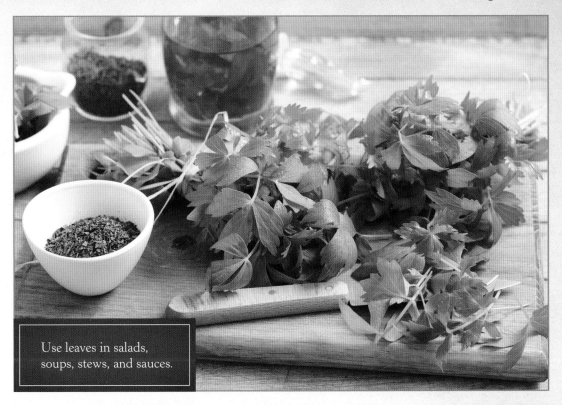

Use leaves in salads, soups, stews, and sauces.

Cultivation: Lovage likes moist, rich, acidic soil. It will grow in full sun or partial shade. Because it dies down in winter, mark its place in the fall to avoid digging the roots and damaging the plant.

Propagation: Sow seeds in late summer; divide in autumn or early spring.

Uses: Herbalists have recommended lovage to increase urine flow, reduce gas and bowel pain, and treat sore throat, kidney stones, and irregular menstruation. Lovage also is used to treat stomachaches, headaches, obesity, and boils. The hot tea induces sweating.

The taste of lovage's leaves, stems, and seeds resembles that of celery but is much sharper. Dried and powdered, they make a tasty addition to herbal salt substitutes. Stems may be cooked, puréed, candied, or eaten raw like celery. Add seeds to pickling brines, cheeses, salad dressings, potatoes, tomatoes, chicken, poultry stuffings, and rice. It also flavors some alcoholic beverages.

Lovage is sometimes used medicinally, but its most common use is as an addition to foods or condiments. The food industry uses lovage essential oil.

Part used: Leaves, stems, seeds

Preservation: Harvest fresh leaves as needed. Pick for later use just before the plant begins to bloom. Blanch whole leaves and freeze, or mince and freeze in cubes. Or you can dry lovage by hanging the stems in bundles. Pick seed heads when they turn brown. Hang them upside-down in paper bags to catch seeds.

Precautions: Do not use lovage if you are pregnant or have any kidney problems.

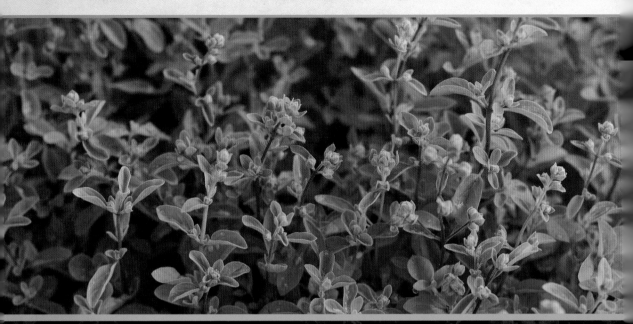

Marjoram

Perennial (often grown as an Annual)

Botanical Name: *Origanum majorana* or *Majorana hortensis*

Family: Lamiaceae (Labiatae)

Height: 1 ft.

Spread: 8 in.

Description: Marjoram is a bushy, spreading, fairly hardy perennial that is grown as an annual in freezing climates. It produces small, oval, gray-green, velvety leaves and knotlike shapes that blossom into tiny white or pink flowers from August through September. The herb makes an attractive potted plant that may be brought inside when temperatures fall. Native to southwest Asia, marjoram has become naturalized in Mediterranean regions and is cultivated widely in North America.

Ease of care: Easy

Cultivation: Like its cousin oregano (*Origanum vulgare*), marjoram likes average to sandy, well-drained alkaline soil and full sun. If your winters are severe, grow marjoram as an annual or in pots that may be brought indoors. If you keep it outdoors, shelter it from the cold.

Propagation: Sow seed indoors a few weeks before the last frost and transplant outdoors after the soil has warmed; take cuttings in spring.

Uses: The Greeks knew marjoram as "joy of the mountains" and used it as a remedy for sadness. Herbalists have prescribed marjoram to treat asthma, increase sweating, lower fevers, encourage menstruation, and, especially, relieve indigestion. European singers preserved their voices with marjoram tea sweetened with honey. The herb has antioxidant and antifungal properties. Recent studies show marjoram inhibits several viruses, including the herpesvirus. Marjoram gargles and steam treatments relieve sinus congestion and hay fever. A massage oil made from marjoram helps relieve muscle and menstrual cramps. The diluted essential oil can be rubbed into sore gums, in place of clove oil. Aromatherapists use the scent to relax the mind, induce sleep, and even relieve grief.

An infusion added to the bath helps relieve aches, pains, and congestion. Marjoram's antiseptic properties make it a good facial cleanser, and it has been used in cosmetic facial waters. Marjoram freshens linen drawers, and you can add it to potpourri and sachets. Dried flowers may be used in crafts and arrangements. The herb dyes wool shades of green and purple, but the color is not long-lasting.

Marjoram can be made into tea, but by far, the most common way to use it is in cooking. It is also available as an essential oil that can be diluted in vegetable oil and applied to the skin. A couple drops of essential oil can be added to a bath or steam.

Part used: Leaves

Preservation: Snip fresh leaves as needed. Harvest leaves just before flowering and hang them to dry.

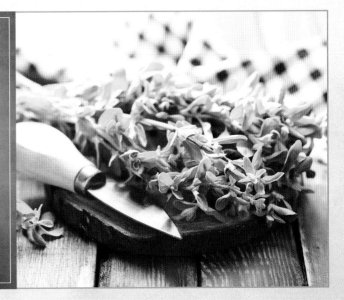

Marjoram tastes like a mild oregano with a hint of balsam. Add leaves to salads, beef, veal, lamb, roasted poultry, fish, and vegetables such as carrots, cauliflower, eggplant, mushrooms, parsnips, potatoes, squash, and tomatoes. The herb also complements stews, marinades, dressings, butters, oils, vinegars, and cheese spreads. Its antioxidant properties are so potent they have been shown to be excellent food preservatives.

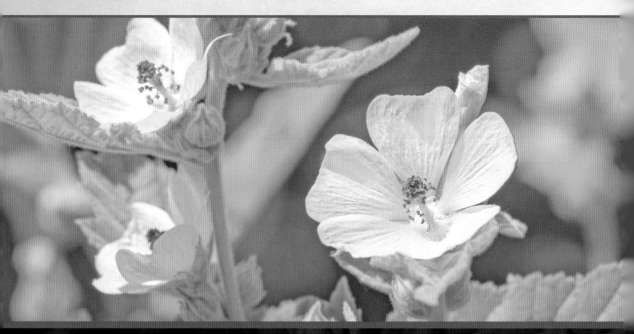

Marshmallow

Perennial

Botanical Name: *Althea officinalis*

Family: Malvaceae

Height: 4 ft.

Spread: 2 ft.

Description: Marshmallow produces a tapering, woody taproot and woolly stems with several spreading, leafy branches. Flowers, pink to pale blue, appear from July through September. Marshmallow is native to Europe and naturalized in eastern North America. It's found in moist woods, salt marshes, and damp land near the sea.

Ease of care: Easy

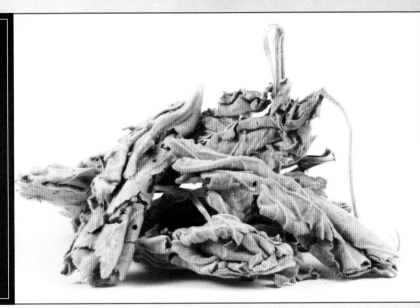

A mixture of dried marshmallow leaves is combined as a tea with herbs such as elecampane, licorice, and mullein to treat coughs and sore throats.

Cultivation: All mallows like full sun to partial shade and moist to wet, light, neutral soil. Mallows are hardy plants that will tolerate hot, dry summers and cold winters.

Propagation: Sow seeds in the fall in moderate climates. Seedlings grow rapidly the first year and should produce blooms by the summer of the second year. Take cuttings or divide in autumn.

Uses: Yes, those popular campfire confections originated with these lovely plants. The Greeks used marshmallow to treat wounds, toothaches, coughing, and insect stings. The Romans valued marshmallow roots and leaves for their laxative properties. And during the Renaissance, marshmallow was used extensively to treat sore throats, stomach problems, and even venereal diseases. Marshmallow is a wonderful demulcent that soothes digestive tract inflammations and irritations; it helps heal stomach ulcers. It is also used in formulas to treat urinary and prostate infections and inflammations. It enhances immunity by stimulating white blood cells. Applied as a poultice, it helps to heal cuts and bruises. The roots are sometimes used in salves and poultices.

In the kitchen, add uncooked young tops and tender leaves to spring salads, or fry roots with butter and onions.

Use roots for teas, pills, or tinctures. Drink 1 or more cups of tea or take up to 2 teaspoons (8 droppers full) of tincture per day of marshmallow. It is usually mixed with other herbs such as saw palmetto, hydrangea, nettle root, and horsetail to treat an enlarged prostate or with uva ursi, horsetail, plantain, and hydrangea to treat urinary infection. To make a marshmallow poultice, mash or blend the fresh root and add enough cold water to form a gooey gel with a paste-like consistency. Apply the mixture directly to the skin.

Part used: Leaves, flowers, roots

Preservation: Gather flowers after they bloom. Collect taproots in autumn from plants at least two years old. Remove lateral rootlets, wash, peel off corky bark, and dry in slices.

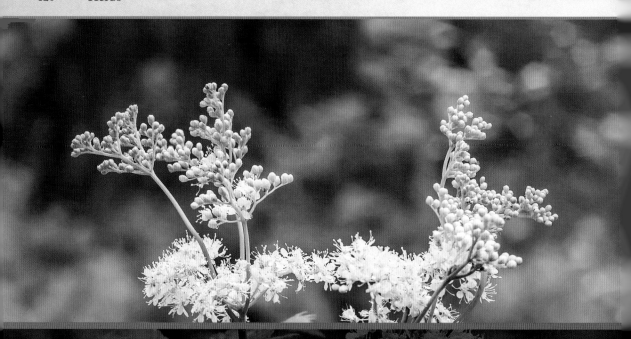

Meadowsweet

Perennial

Botanical Name: *Filipendula ulmaria*

Family: Rosaceae

Height: To 6 ft., in flower

Spread: 2 ft.

Description: Meadowsweet produces elmlike leaves and large clusters of small white flowers, which bloom throughout summer and smell faintly of almonds. Also known as queen of the meadow, the herb grows wild in Europe and Asia and has been naturalized in North America, from Newfoundland to Ohio. You will find it growing in marshes, along stream banks, and in forests and meadows.

Ease of care: Easy

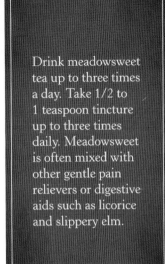
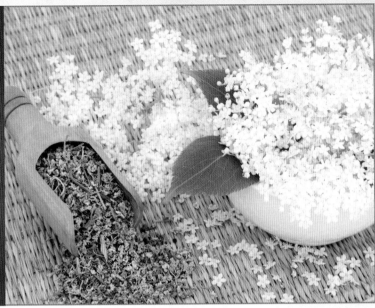

Drink meadowsweet tea up to three times a day. Take 1/2 to 1 teaspoon tincture up to three times daily. Meadowsweet is often mixed with other gentle pain relievers or digestive aids such as licorice and slippery elm.

Cultivation: Meadowsweet prefers rich, moist, well-drained soil and partial shade.

Propagation: Grow from seed or divide the roots of older plants in the spring or fall. It needs plenty of water to bloom.

Uses: The next time you take an aspirin, you can thank meadowsweet. It was from this former strewing herb that 19th-century German chemists developed the popular over-the-counter remedy. Meadowsweet's flower buds contain the pain-reliever salicin, from which researchers derived salicylic acid, aspirin's main component. Meadowsweet's ability to reduce pain is not as marked as aspirin's concentrated compounds, but the plant does not produce aspirin's main side effect: upset stomach. The herb is even used to ease the discomfort of stomach ulcers. It prevents excess acid in the stomach and is one of the best herbal treatments for heartburn.

Meadowsweet has been prescribed to treat headache, arthritis, menstrual cramps, stomach cramps and gas, low-grade fever, and inflammation. It also contains a chemical that fights diarrhea-causing bacteria. Meadowsweet promotes excretion of uric acid, so it is used to treat gout (a condition of excess uric acid) and some types of kidney stones. As an antiseptic diuretic, it is used for urinary tract infections. New research shows that meadowsweet may help prevent blood clots that can trigger heart attacks. Other studies indicate that the salicin in meadowsweet reduces blood sugar levels and may have use in managing diabetes.

Part used: Flowers

Preservation: Harvest flower tops when the plant is in bloom. Dry or tincture.

Precautions: There are no known contra-indications for meadowsweet; however, aspirin has been associated with birth defects and may trigger the fatal Reye syndrome if given to children with colds, flu, or chicken pox, so avoid giving meadowsweet to sick youngsters, until it is proved a safe alternative to aspirin.

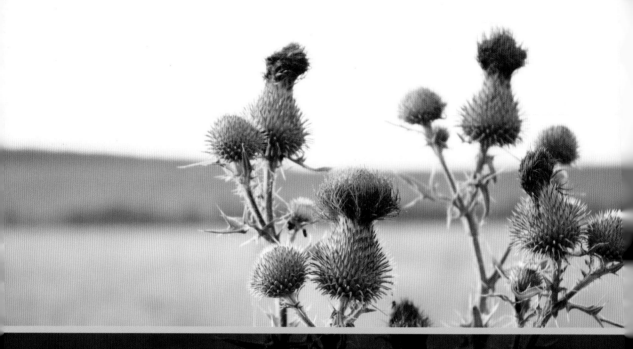

Milk Thistle

Annual or Biennial

Botanical Name: *Silybum marianum*

Family: Asteraceae (Compositae)

Height: To 3 ft., in flower

Spread: To 3 ft.

Description: Milk thistle leaves are large, shiny, and spiny. Violet-purple flowers appear from late summer to early autumn. Milk thistle is native to central and western Europe and has become naturalized elsewhere. It is often found on dry, rocky or stony soils in wastelands and fields, and along roads.

Ease of care: Easy

Cultivation: Milk thistle prefers sun and well-drained soil.

Propagation: The herb grows easily from seed.

Uses: Legend has it that milk thistle sprang from the milk of the Virgin Mary, and for centuries, herbalists have recommended it for increasing milk in nursing mothers. But the herb's primary use in modern times is in detoxifying and nourishing the liver. The flavonoids in milk thistle repair damaged liver cells, stimulate production of new cells, and protect existing cells. In Europe, victims of *Amanita* mushroom poisoning who received preparations made from a compound in milk thistle survived. This is remarkable because *Amanita* mushrooms are normally considered deadly—most people who eat them die of liver failure. Herbalists prescribe milk thistle to treat jaundice, hepatitis, cirrhosis, and other liver conditions caused by alcohol abuse. Benefits are noted in about two weeks.

Milk thistle contains essential oils, tyramine, histamine, and a flavonoid called silymarine. Milk thistle has antioxidant properties and counteracts some of the detrimental effects of environmental toxins. A bitter tonic, the leaves stimulate bile production—it has been prescribed to improve appetite and assist digestion. Once cultivated widely as a nutritious culinary herb, young milk thistle leaves may be eaten as a salad or potherb. To eat the leaves, cut off their sharp edges with scissors and steam. Serve as you would spinach.

Drink a milk thistle tea up to three times a day. Take up to 1/2 teaspoon (2 droppers full) of tincture up to three times a day, or take milk thistle in pill form.

Part used: Seeds, leaves, and shoots

Preservation: Gather shoots and leaves in spring, seeds in late summer when ripe. Dry or tincture the seeds.

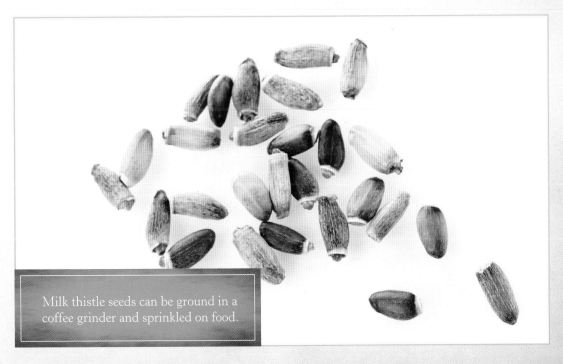

Milk thistle seeds can be ground in a coffee grinder and sprinkled on food.

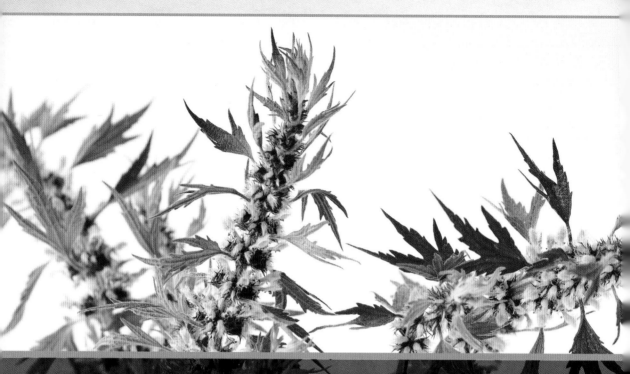

Motherwort

Perennial

Botanical Name: *Leonurus cardiaca*

Family: Lamiaceae (Labiatae)

Height: 4 ft.

Spread: 1 ft.; may become invasive

Description: Motherwort has stout, square stems tinged with red or violet. Lower leaves are lobed, like those of maple. Upper leaves are narrow and toothed. The plant produces whorls of small, white, pink, or red blooms in summer.

Ease of care: Easy

Cultivation: Motherwort prefers average, well-drained soil and full sun but will tolerate most conditions.

Propagation: Sow seed in the spring; thin seedlings to 12 inches.

Uses: As its name implies, motherwort is useful for treating conditions associated with childbirth. The herb contains a chemical called leonurine, which encourages uterine contractions. Motherwort is used as a uterine tonic before and after childbirth. It has also been used for centuries to regulate the menstrual cycle, to promote the flow of mother's milk, and to treat menopausal complaints.

Motherwort is a mild relaxing agent often recommended by herbalists to reduce anxiety and depression and treat nervousness, insomnia, heart palpitations, and rapid heart rate. Russian studies show that motherwort is good for hypertension because it relaxes blood vessels and calms nerves. Motherwort injections have been shown to prevent formation of blood clots, which improves blood flow and reduces risk of heart attack, stroke, and other diseases. Motherwort is also useful for headache, insomnia, vertigo, and delirium from fever. It is sometimes used to relieve asthma, bronchitis, and other lung problems, usually mixed with mullein and other lung herbs.

Drink up to 4 cups of motherwort tea a day. It is bitter; you may wish to mix it with other herbs. It is often taken with other women's tonics such as red raspberry or heart tonics such as hawthorn. Take up to 1 teaspoon (4 droppers full) of tincture a day.

Part used: Leaves

Preservation: Harvest leaves after flowers bloom; dry or tincture.

Precautions: Don't use motherwort if you have clotting problems or take medication to thin your blood. Avoid motherwort if you are pregnant, unless a health professional recommends its use. Some people may develop a rash after handling motherwort.

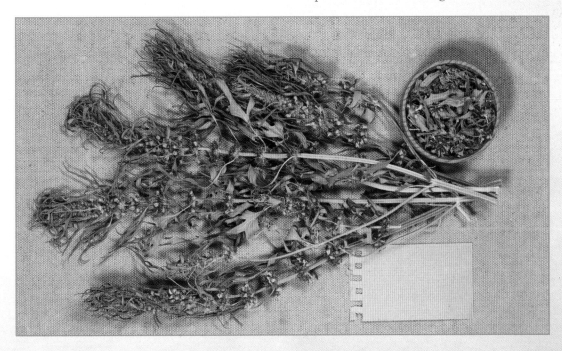

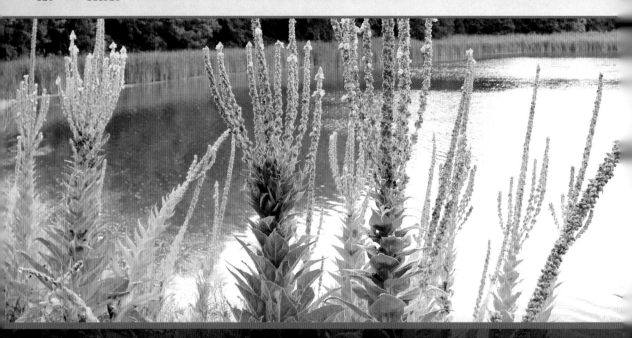

Mullein

Biennial

Botanical Name: *Verbascum thapsus*

Family: Scrophulariaceae

Height: To 7 ft. in full flower; the leaves, to 8 in.

Spread: 2–3 ft.

Description: Mullein is a common plant, often found along roads and in untended fields. The herb's leaves have soft, fine hairs, which irritate the mucous membranes of animals that attempt to eat them. The woolly leaves also protect the herb from moisture loss and insects. Mullein's round, fibrous stem is sturdy and downy and produces bright yellow flowers from midsummer to early autumn. Dried, the flowers exude a very faint, honeylike scent.

Ease of care: Easy

Cultivation: Don't try to grow mullein indoors. It prefers open spaces. Mullein likes rich soil but will grow in poor soil in dry wastelands. Thin or transplant to 3 feet.

Propagation: Sow seeds in spring or summer. Mullein readily self-seeds.

Uses: According to Homer, mullein was given to Ulysses to protect him from Circe's sorcery. For centuries, mullein was considered

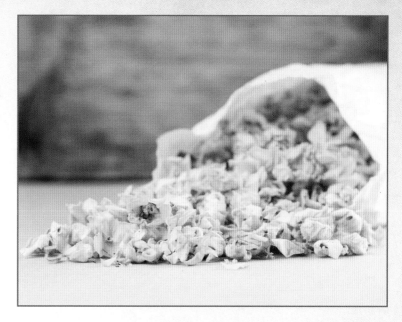

an amulet against witches and evil spirits. Also called Aaron's rod, candlewick plant, hag's taper, and velvet dock, the plant has many uses—from medicinal to household. Citing just one example, the dried stems were dipped in suet and burned as torches.

For centuries, mullein's leaves have been used to heal lung conditions. Herbalists once even recommended that patients with lung diseases smoke dried, crumbled mullein leaves. Ayurvedic physicians prescribed mullein to treat coughs. And colonists considered mullein so valuable they brought it with them to America, where Indians eventually adopted it for treating coughs, bronchitis, and asthma.

Contemporary herbalists still recommend internal use of mullein leaves to treat colds, sore throat, and coughs. The flowers and leaves reduce inflammation in the urinary and digestive tract and treat colitis, intestinal bleeding, and diarrhea. The fresh flower infused alone or with garlic in olive oil makes an ear oil for pain and inflammation associated with an earache.

The leaves make good tinder, and the dried tops can be used in flower arrangements. Flower infusions are employed in creams, facial steams, and shampoos to soothe skin and brighten fair hair.

You can take mullein leaves in pill, tincture, or tea form. Use up to a few cups of tea or a teaspoon of tincture (4 droppers full) a day. Mullein is often combined with other herbs that treat lung conditions, such as elecampane.

Part used: Flowers, leaves

Preservation: Harvest leaves during mullein's first growing season and flowers as soon as they open. The flower stalk appears the second year. To preserve mullein, remove the green parts from the flowers, then dry the flowers gently without artificial heat. Be careful not to lose the yellow color, which is part of the healing substance. Leaves may be dried as well.

Precautions: The fine hairs on the leaves irritate some people's skin and cause a rash.

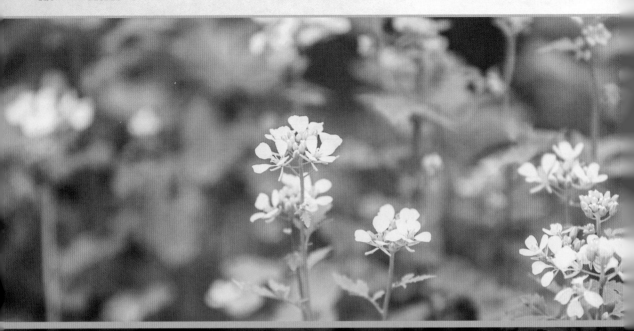

Mustard

Perennial

Botanical Name: *Brassica alba*

Family: Cruciferae

Height: To 2 ft.

Spread: 1 ft.

Description: You'll recognize species of the large mustard family by their strong smell and four-petaled flowers. Mustard flowers are small and yellow, and the petals resemble a Maltese cross. Lower leaves are pinnately lobed or coarsely toothed; upper leaves are not as lobed. The plant flowers in early summer. Mustards grow just about everywhere. These are hardy plants. White mustard grows wild throughout the world and has many cousins, including cabbage, broccoli, and turnips.

Ease of care: Easy

Cultivation: Plant mustard seeds 1/8 inch deep in a sunny spot, where the soil is average to poor and well drained. Yellow mustard tolerates heavy soil conditions better than black mustard. Thin seedlings to about 9 inches apart. Mustard prefers heavy feeding: Regularly add well-rotted manure or compost to the soil. Mustard supposedly stimulates growth of beans, grapes, and fruit trees. It is said to keep flea beetles away from collards. Mustard also releases a chemical in the soil that inhibits cyst nematodes and prevents root rot and also many other plants from growing near it.

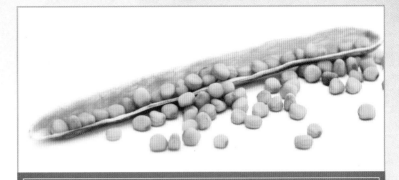

Winnow seeds from pods by rubbing them in the palm of your hand.

Propagation: To grow mustard for its leaves, sow seeds at several intervals from spring through early fall. If you're growing mustard for its seeds, sow in spring or late summer. Once established, it will easily self-sow; it can even become a garden pest.

Uses: You haven't really tasted mustard until you've made it yourself. To make mustard from seeds, boil 1/3 cup cider vinegar, 2/3 cup cider, 2 tablespoons honey, 1/8 tablespoon turmeric, and up to 1 teaspoon salt. While hot, combine with 1/4 cup ground mustard seeds. Blend in a food processor. After the mixture is smooth, add 1 tablespoon olive oil. This recipe makes 1 1/4 cups of mustard.

Mustard has many medicinal uses, too. If you're old enough, you may even remember getting a mustard plaster when you had a cold. Mustard seeds warm the skin and open the lungs to make breathing easier.

Mustard plasters may also relieve rheumatism, toothache, sore muscles, and arthritis. Its chief constituent, mustard oil, gives it its heat and flavor. These constituents also make mustard an appetite stimulate and a powerful irritant. Mustard in small doses improves digestion. Young leaves are vitamin-rich additions to salads, or they can be boiled with onions and salt pork.

To make a poultice, mix powdered seeds with an equal amount of flour and enough water to form a paste. Spread mustard plaster on a cloth and place the cloth, poultice side down, on the skin. Leave on about 20 minutes. Remove if the poultice becomes uncomfortable. Wash affected area.

Part used: Leaves, seeds

Preservation: Harvest leaves for salads when they are young and tender. Harvest seeds when pods have turned brown but before they split open. Spread plants on a tray. Within a couple of weeks the seeds should ripen. Store whole or ground mustard seed in tightly covered jars.

Precautions: Consuming large quantities of mustard seed may cause vomiting. Don't leave mustard plasters on too long or they may blister skin.

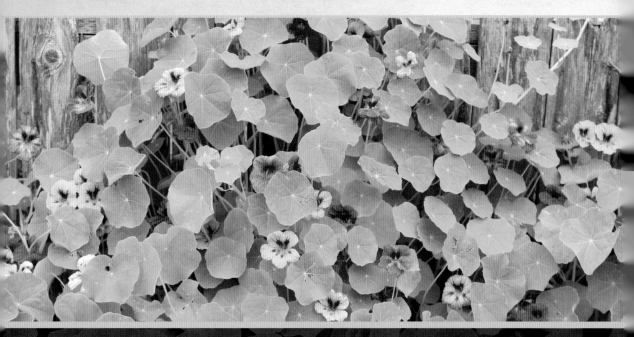

Nasturtium

Annual

Botanical Name: *Tropaeolum majus*

Family: Tropaeolaceae

Height: 1 ft., bush; 5–10 ft., vines

Spread: 1 1/2 ft., bush; vines ramble

Description: Nasturtiums produce distinctive, blue-green circular leaves on fleshy stems. The plants come in a variety of types, ranging from compact bushes to spreading vines. They produce large, attractive blooms that range from pale yellow, pink, and apricot to deep, rich gold, orange, and burgundy. Nasturtiums are native to South America and widely cultivated elsewhere.

Ease of care: Easy

Cultivation: Nasturtiums like full sun to partial shade in average to poor, moist soil. They are said to repel whiteflies, cabbage pests, and squash bugs. But they attract aphids, so be on the lookout for these insects. The plant flowers throughout summer until the first frost. Beautiful ornamental plants, nasturtiums make an eye-catching addition to any garden. Vines are great in hanging planters, in window boxes, or on trellises and fences.

Propagation: Seeds are large. Sow them in late spring in any spot that can use bright color and where vines have a place to climb.

Uses: Spanish conquerors brought nasturtiums from Peru to Spain. Soon these lovely flowering herbs spread across the continent. Nasturtium leaves have a peppery flavor and make good additions to salads. Flower buds may be cured in vinegar and used like capers. They can also be stuffed with cream cheese or blended with butter. Pull off the individual petals to add color and flavor to a salad. The natural antibiotic in nasturtiums is effective even against some microorganisms that have built up a resistance to antibiotic drugs. The leaves and flowers fight infections of the lung and reproductive and urinary tracts. To relieve itching skin, try rubbing the juice of the fresh plant on the skin.

Nasturtiums are medicinal when eaten. You can use them as a tincture; however, they are seldom used in this form. Sometimes the leaves are added to herb teas. One tasty way to use nasturtium is to make an herbal vinegar to use on salads.

Part used: Leaves, flowers

Preservation: Harvest fresh leaves and flowers as needed. Pickle unripe seeds in vinegar and use them in salads.

Precautions: Large amounts of the seeds act as a strong laxative (purgative).

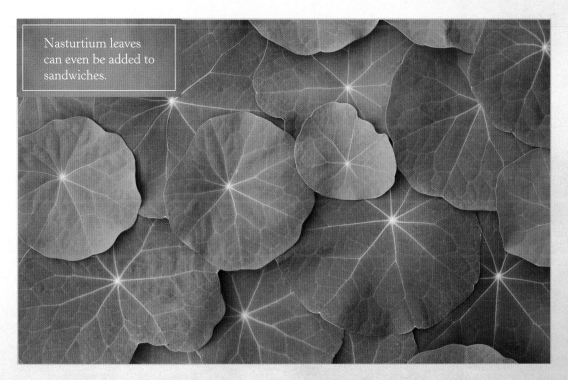

Nasturtium leaves can even be added to sandwiches.

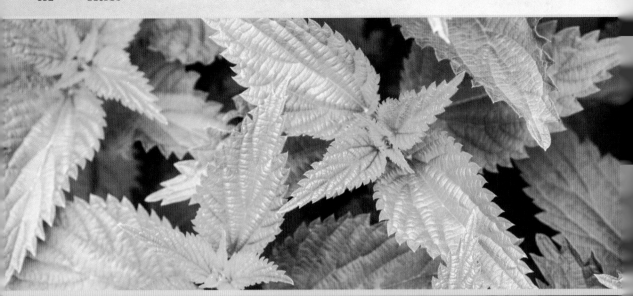

Nettle

Perennial

Botanical Name: *Urtica dioica*

Family: Urticaceae

Height: 3–6 ft.

Spread: 1–2 ft.

Description: Brush against a bushy nettle plant and you'll feel as if you've been stung by bees. The herb's single stalk forms dark-green, saw-toothed leaves, which are covered with tiny "hairs" containing formic acid, a substance that causes pain if it comes in contact with your skin. Nettle's small, greenish flowers appear in clusters from July through September. The herb is native to Europe and Asia and widely naturalized. In North America it ranges from Newfoundland to Ontario, west to Colorado, and south to the Carolinas. You'll find nettle in weedy places, often near water.

Ease of care: Easy

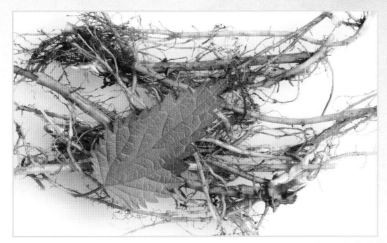

inflammation. Nettle treats eczema and skin rashes, increases mother's milk, slightly lowers blood sugar, and decreases profuse menstruation.

Nettle is so versatile that it has been used for centuries as a spring tonic to improve general health. The herb is rich in flavonoids and vital nutrients, including vitamins D, C, and A as well as minerals, such as iron, calcium, phosphorus, and magnesium. Thus, nettle has been used to treat malnutrition, anemia, and rickets. Hair shampoos and conditioners often include nettle because it is said to benefit the scalp and encourage hair growth.

Cultivation: Nettle prefers average to rich, moist soil and full sun to partial shade. Gardeners like it in their gardens because nettle may stimulate growth and production of essential oils in companion plants. Nettle also hosts several beneficial insects that prey on harmful pests. But it can be very invasive. To prevent this, cut it way back when harvesting before it goes to seed. You may need to do this several times every summer.

Propagation: Nettle grows from seeds dispersed in spring, or you can produce new plants by dividing in spring or fall.

Uses: The Anglo-Saxons named nettle after their word for "needle." During the Bronze Age, fabric was woven from nettle. As recently as World War I, Germans wove nettle fabric when cotton supplies were low.

Nettle was once used to reduce arthritic pains and uric acid in joints and tissues (excess uric acid causes gout, a painful inflammatory condition). Nettle improves circulation and treats asthma. It is a light laxative; nettle tea has also been prescribed for intestinal weakness, diarrhea, and malnutrition. Nettle is a diuretic useful for treating bladder problems. Several studies demonstrated that the root successfully reduces prostate

Nettle loses its sting when cooked, dried, or ground. It is a healthy and tasty addition to scrambled eggs, pasta dishes, casseroles, and soups. Young shoots may be steamed then tossed in salads or eaten like kale or spinach. You also may juice nettle and drink it alone or combine it with other fruit or vegetable juices. Nettle leaves dye wool shades of yellow and green.

Drink 2 to 6 cups a day. Take 1 to 2 teaspoons (4 to 8 droppers full) of tincture per day. Drink 1 to 2 ounces of juice per day, or eat nettle as a vegetable. Nettle is often mixed with different herbs in a variety of medicinal preparations.

Part used: Root, leaves

Preservation: Tincture fresh or dried nettle.

Precautions: Wear gloves to pick nettles. Ingesting large amounts of older nettle plants may irritate the kidneys.

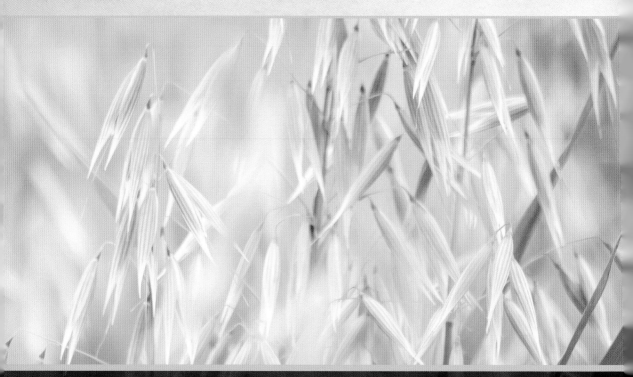

Oats

Annual

Botanical Name: *Avena sativa*

Family: Gramineae

Height: 2–4 ft.

Spread: 1 in.

Description: The grass produces a fibrous root and a hollow jointed stem with narrow, flat, pale-green leaves. The grain is "hairy" and grooved. Oats are native to southern Europe and eastern Asia. They are widely cultivated as a food.

Ease of care: Easy

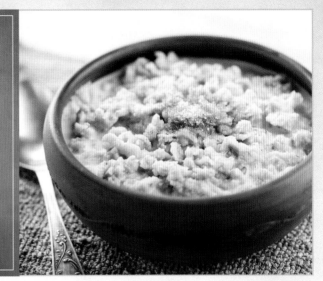

Is there anyone who has not eaten oatmeal? This ubiquitous and nourishing cereal contains starches, proteins, vitamins, minerals, and dietary fiber nutritionists recommend we consume each day. Several clinical trials have found that regular consumption of oat bran reduces blood cholesterol levels in just one month. High-fiber diets may also reduce risk of colon and rectal cancer. Oats contain the alkaloid gramine, which has been credited with mild sedative properties.

Cultivation: Widely cultivated for their nourishing grain, oats can also be grown in an herb garden.

Propagation: Sow seed in spring.

Uses: The oat seed is used in two different phases of its growth: in its fresh, milky stage and as a grain once the seed is ripe and dried. In its milky stage, oat tincture has been prescribed for nerve disorders and as a uterine tonic. Researchers found that fresh oats have some value in treating addiction and reducing nicotine craving. Fresh, green oats ease the anxiety that often accompanies drug withdrawal. Oat straw is sometimes made into a high-mineral tea.

Oatmeal has been used topically to heal wounds and various skin rashes. With their demulcent and soothing qualities, oats are found in soaps and bath and body products. Oatmeal baths and poultices are wonderful for soothing dry, flaky skin or alleviating itching from poison oak and chicken pox. Used in the bath, oatmeal makes a good facial scrub and helps clear up skin problems.

Take 1/4 to 3/4 teaspoon (1 to 3 droppers full) a day of a tincture of fresh oats. Make a paste by adding water to ground oats. You can easily grind them in a coffee grinder or a food processor. For a bath, put fine-ground oats in a porous bag and place in bath water. This bag can be used to scrub the body in place of soap for people who are sensitive to soap. Oat straw tea is often combined with other high-mineral herbs, such as nettles. The fresh oats are used with other nervous system herbs, such as St. John's wort.

Part used: Grain, fresh berry, and shaft (oat straw)

Preservation: Gather fresh oats and oat straw in the spring and the oat berry in the late summer. Oat straw and whole dried oat groats may be dried. The fresh oat seed must be fresh-tinctured—once it is dried, it loses some of its medicinal properties.

Precautions: Most people tolerate oats well, but some people, especially those with bowel disorders, may experience discomfort after suddenly increasing fiber consumption. Always drink plenty of liquids after eating fibrous foods. If you have an intolerance to gluten-containing grains, don't eat oats.

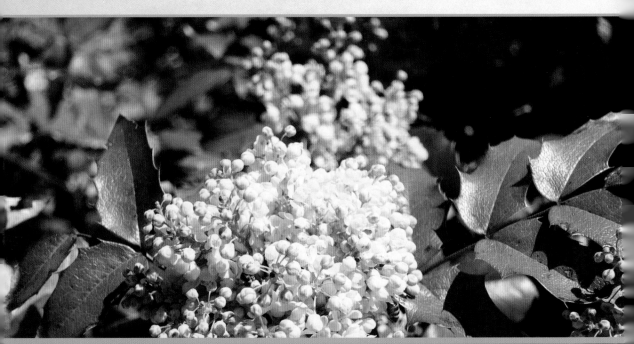

Oregon Grape

Perennial

Botanical Name: *Berberis aquifolium*

Family: Berberidaceae

Height: 3–6 ft.

Spread: To 4 ft.

Description: An evergreen shrub, Oregon grape produces dense, oblong leaves with prickly edges similar to those of holly. The dark green leaves turn bronze, crimson, or purple in fall. Tiny flowers are bright yellow in spring; the inner bark of the rhizome is also bright yellow. The tree produces deep purple berries. Oregon grape is found in coniferous forests throughout the American Northwest and Canada.

Ease of care: Easy

Cultivation: Oregon grape prefers well-drained, humusy soil and full sun. The plant hosts wheat rust fungus but is immune to the disease. Oregon grape may suffer from leaf spot and powdery mildew.

Propagation: Take cuttings in midsummer and set out new plants the following spring. Collect berries in fall and plant seeds in spring.

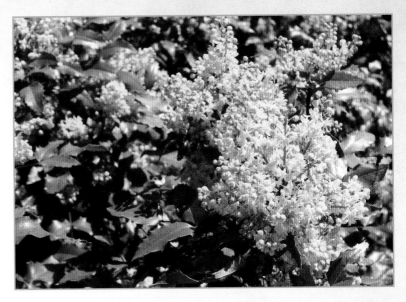

Uses: Oregon grape's prime constituent, the alkaloid berberine, improves blood flow to the liver and stimulates bile to aid digestion. Thus, Oregon grape root may be used to boost liver function and treat jaundice, hepatitis, poor intestinal tone and function, and gastrointestinal debility. Berberine effectively kills *Giardia* and *Candida* organisms and several other intestinal parasites, which are responsible for intestinal upsets and vaginal yeast infections. Oregon grape root is useful to treat serious cases of diarrhea and digestive tract infection. Oregon grape is also useful for treating colds, flu, and numerous other infections. In the laboratory, it's been shown to kill or suppress the growth of several disease-causing microbes. Oregon grape's berberine content makes it a good eye wash, douche, or skin cleanser for infections. The tincture is used to treat eczema, acne, herpes, and psoriasis.

High in vitamin C, the berries may be eaten raw or cooked in jam. Berries are also used to flavor jelly, wine, and soups. They have been used in folk medicine and seem to have some of the same medicinal properties as the root, but they are probably not as potent. Oregon grape root and bark dye wool yellow and tan; fruits impart a purplish blue color.

You can drink up to 3 cups of tea a day, although due to the bitter taste, you will probably want to mix it with other herbs or take the herb as a tincture. Take 1/2 to 1 teaspoon of the tincture (2 to 4 droppers full) up to three times a day. For an eye wash, make a strong tea (2 teaspoons of Oregon grape per cup of water) and strain carefully through a coffee filter before using in an eye cup.

Part used: Root (the medicine is in the yellow area under the outer root bark), berries

Preservation: Dig roots in fall, and dry in a paper bag.

Precautions: Oregon grape stimulates liver function, so if you have liver disease, use only under the care of a health practitioner. Avoid it if you are pregnant. Otherwise, use the herb for two to three weeks, abstain for several weeks, and resume if necessary.

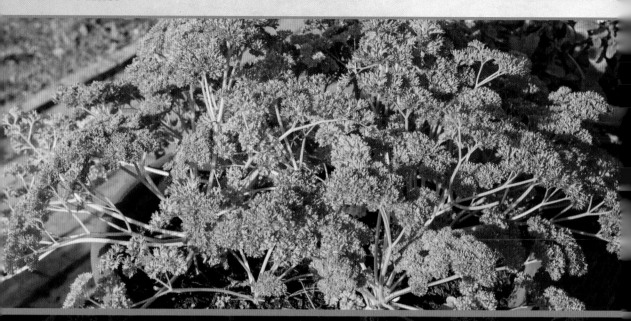

Parsley

Biennial (often grown as an Annual)

Botanical Name: *Petroselinum crispum*

Family: Apiaceae (Umbelliferae)

Height: 2–3 ft., in flower

Spread: 8 in.

Description: Parsley is often grown as an annual to obtain fresh-tasting leaves. The herb's attractive, rich-green, dense leaves form a rosette base, and the plant produces tiny, greenish-yellow flowers in early summer. Parsley comes in two forms: curly and Italian. The latter has flat leaves and is stronger-flavored than the curly variety. Curly parsley makes a nice edging plant, and both varieties can be grown in pots indoors. Parsley grows wild in many parts of the world and is cultivated throughout the temperate world.

Ease of care: Easy

Cultivation: Parsley prefers full sun or partial shade in a moist, rich soil. Parsley is said to repel asparagus beetles.

Propagation: Soak seeds in warm water for several hours to speed germination. Sow seeds in the garden once the soil is warm in spring. The seeds often take many weeks to germinate. Parsley is difficult to transplant unless small.

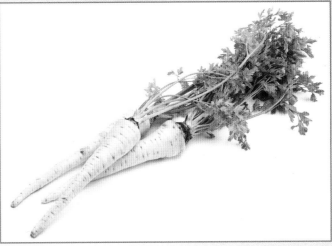

Uses: You may think of parsley as a "throw-away" herb. It is universally used as a garnish that often goes uneaten. But if you discard this natural breath sweetener, you'll be wasting a powerhouse of vitamins and minerals. Parsley contains vitamins A and C (more than an orange), and small amounts of several B vitamins, calcium, and iron. The leaves and root have diuretic properties and are used to treat bladder infections. Parsley's strong odor derives from its essential oils, one of which, apiol, has been extracted for medicinal uses. It is used in pharmaceutical drugs to treat some kidney ailments. Parsley seeds, or a compound in them, is used in some pharmaceutical preparations to treat urinary tract disorders. Another of parsley's compounds reduces inflammation and is a free radical scavenger, eliminating these destructive elements. It also stimulates the appetite and increases circulation to the digestive organs. The root has more medicinal properties than the leaves.

Parsley's clean flavor blends with most foods and is often found in ethnic cuisines, including those of the Middle East, France, Belgium, Switzerland, Japan, Spain, and England. Parsley complements most meats and poultry and is a good addition to vegetable dishes, soups, and stews. It is always an ingredient in the famous *bouquet garni* used by cooks throughout the Western world. To make white sauce, the stems are used instead of the leaves to impart less color.

Add parsley to foods to obtain its benefits. Parsley can also be taken in tea, tincture, and pill form. Take the root or leaves in tea or 1/4 teaspoon (1 dropper full) of tincture a day. Commercially, parsley root is used mostly for its diuretic properties and is almost always mixed with other herbs. Occasionally, parsley is added to herbal teas for the treatment of urinary tract problems.

Part used: Leaves, stems, seeds, root

Preservation: Snip leaves as needed and use fresh. Hang-dry parsley or freeze. To prepare the roots, wash and cut them into small pieces while they are fresh and pliable. Dry on a screen in a warm place.

Precautions: Avoid the root, seeds, and large amounts of the leaves if you're pregnant. Also avoid the root and seeds if you have kidney problems. Parsley is fine to eat in foods, however.

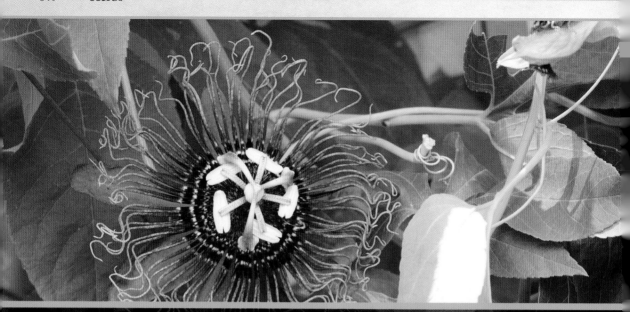

Passion Flower

Perennial

Botanical Name: *Passiflora incarnata*

Family: Passifloraceae

Height: 25–30 ft.

Spread: Creeping vine

Description: Passion flower produces coiling tendrils and showy, colorful blossoms with white or lavender petals and a brilliant pink or purple corona. Flowers appear from early to late summer. The plant produces three to five toothed, lobed leaves and a berry with thin yellow skin and a sweet, succulent pulp. Passion flower is native from Florida to Texas and may be found as far north as Missouri. The herb also is abundant in South America. Passion flower grows in full sun to partially shaded, dry areas, in thickets, along fences, and at the edge of wooded areas.

Ease of care: Moderate

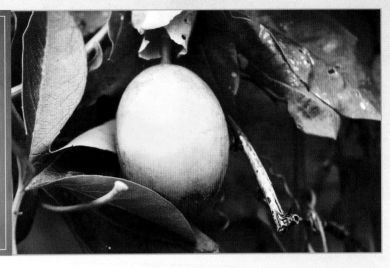

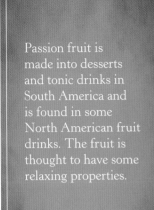

Passion fruit is made into desserts and tonic drinks in South America and is found in some North American fruit drinks. The fruit is thought to have some relaxing properties.

Cultivation: Passion flower prefers deep, well-drained soil, plenty of water, and some shade. Revitalize the soil each spring, replacing the top layer with new topsoil, but don't over-fertilize since very rich soil results in fewer flowers. Prune old branches in late winter and early spring to get better blossoms. The herb is susceptible to thrips and mealybugs. You can also grow passion flower indoors in a large pot, although it won't reach its normal height.

Propagation: Sow seeds in the spring, although they can take years to germinate. Take cuttings in spring or fall. Plants are sold in most nurseries.

Uses: Few herbs have as many religious connections as passion flower. When Spanish explorers discovered the vine growing in South America, they were struck by its elaborate blossoms. Passion flower's five petals and five sepals, they reasoned, represented the 10 faithful apostles. The flower's dramatic corona looked to them like Jesus's crown of thorns. And the herb's five stamens symbolized Christ's five wounds. Curling tendrils reminded them of the cords used to whip Jesus, and the leaves were seen as the hands of his persecutors.

Passion flower's chief medicinal value is as a sedative. The Aztecs used it to promote sleep and relieve pain. Today the flowers are used in numerous pharmaceutical drugs in Europe to treat nervous disorders, heart palpitations, anxiety, and high blood pressure. It has also been prescribed for tension, fatigue, insomnia, and muscle and lung spasms. Unlike most sedative drugs, it has been shown to be nonaddictive, although it is not a strong pain reliever.

Take passion flower as a tea, a tincture, or in pills. A daily dose is 1 to 3 cups of tea or 1/4 to 3/4 teaspoons (1 to 3 droppers full) of tincture. It is often mixed with other sedative herbs, such as valerian, skullcap, and hops.

Part used: Flowers, fruit

Preservation: Gather flowers after they bloom, and dry or tincture.

Precautions: Used in moderation, passion flower is considered safe. Don't use its close relative blue passion flower, which is commonly grown because it is one of the more hardy species.

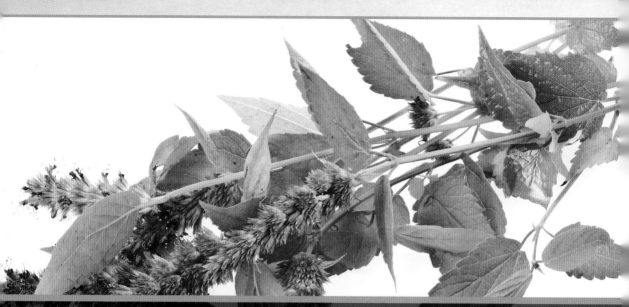

Peppermint

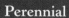

Perennial

Botanical Name: *Mentha piperita*

Family: Lamiaceae (Labiatae)

Height: 2–2 1/2 ft.

Spread: 1 ft.

Description: Peppermint produces dark-green, spear-shaped leaves on stems that arise from an underground network of spreading stems. Though peppermint and spearmint are close relatives, spearmint *(M. spicata)* has green, pointed, somewhat hairy leaves and has a milder, cooler taste. Both plants can become invasive, so plant them in an isolated location, or contain the herbs in a pot. The herb flowers in July and August. Mints are native to Europe and Asia; some varieties are found in South Africa, America, and Australia. They have become naturalized throughout North America, from Canada to Mexico.

Ease of care: Easy

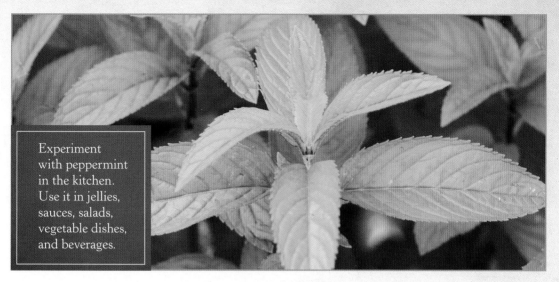

Experiment with peppermint in the kitchen. Use it in jellies, sauces, salads, vegetable dishes, and beverages.

Cultivation: Peppermint likes full sun to partial shade and average, moist soil. Mints are said to repel aphids, flea beetles, and cabbage pests.

Propagation: Take cuttings in midsummer; divide at any time during the growing season.

Uses: You may enjoy peppermint candies, especially after a meal, but this useful plant isn't found just in confections. A carminative and gastric stimulant, promoting the flow of bile to the stomach and aiding digestion, peppermint has been prescribed to treat indigestion, flatulence, colic, and nausea. An antispasmodic, peppermint calms muscles in the digestive tract, reduces colon spasms, and is recommended as a treatment for irritable bowel syndrome and colitis. It also reduces the inflammation of stomach ulcers and colitis. The herb—even its fragrance—eases the pain of headaches. Peppermint's main compound, menthol, is very antiseptic, killing bacteria, viruses, fungi, and parasites, while balancing intestinal flora. Menthol is found in most heating balms, vapor balms, and liniments because of its heating properties.

Peppermint is used to flavor candy, gum, and even dental products and toothpicks. Peppermint makes a good addition to sachets and potpourri. Sniffing peppermint helps clear the sinuses, so it is often used in inhalers. Studies also show that inhaling peppermint stimulates brain waves, increases concentration, and helps keep you awake. Steeped in rosemary vinegar, peppermint helps to control dandruff.

Drink the tasty tea freely. In tinctures, peppermint is most often mixed with other herbs that aid digestion or are relaxing. Take the tea or a few drops of peppermint extract to ease digestion or motion sickness. Use the essential oil in liniments or a vapor balm.

Part used: Leaves

Preservation: Pick shoots in early to middle summer. Hang-dry or freeze.

Precautions: Peppermint is safe to use in moderation. If you have a hiatal hernia, gastroesophageal reflux disease, or chronic heartburn, peppermint could worsen the symptoms.

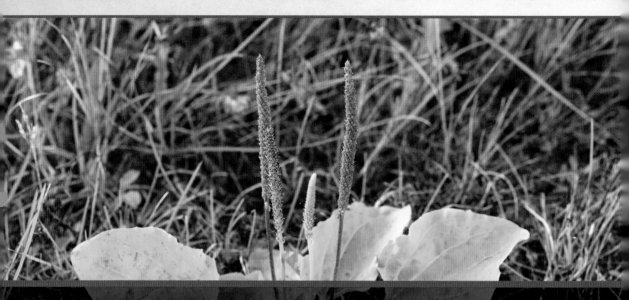

Plantain

Perennial

Botanical Name: *Plantago major*

Family: Plantaginaceae

Height: 1/2–1 1/2 ft.

Spread: To 7 in.

Description: Plantain is native to Europe, but it's probably growing in your own backyard. Hardy and adaptable, plantain has made itself at home throughout the world. American Indians, in fact, called it "white man's foot" because it seemed to follow the European colonists wherever they went. Often you'll see plantain growing along roads, in meadows and, to the chagrin of homeowners, in lawns. *Plantago major* has thick, broad, and oval leaves that form a compact rosette. The even more common *P. lanceolata* has similar leaves, but they are much more narrow. The herb's flowers are very tiny and yellowish-green, appearing from June through September.

Ease of care: Easy

Cultivation: Extremely hardy, plantain thrives in average, well-drained soil in full sun to shade.

Propagation: Sow seed in early spring or fall. The plant grows quickly and self-seeds readily. But before you plant seeds, check your lawn. Chances are plantain already grows there.

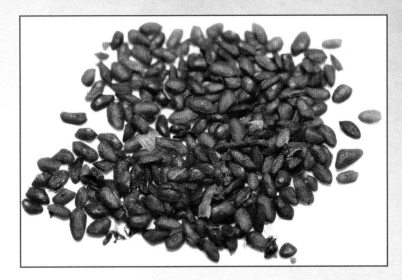

Uses: Don't consider this ubiquitous plant a nuisance. Plantain is a powerful healer and has been used for centuries to treat a variety of ailments. The ancient Saxons, in fact, regarded plantain as one of the essential herbs.

If a bee stings you, apply crushed, fresh plantain leaves to the welt, which will soon disappear. And if you stumble into a patch of poison ivy, you needn't scratch and suffer. Apply a poultice of plantain leaves to relieve your discomfort. Some people, moreover, have been known to chew plantain root to stop the pain of a toothache. A diuretic, the herb is useful for treating urinary problems. Lung disorders, such as asthma and bronchitis, also respond to plantain. Research from India shows that it reduces the symptoms of colds and coughs and relieves the pain and wheezing associated with bronchial problems.

In the kitchen, steam tender young plantain leaves as you would spinach, or eat small amounts fresh in salads, although they are too fibrous for most people's tastes. The seeds are edible. Add small amounts to other grains to increase protein. The species *P. psyllium* is a popular laxative; it is used, as is *P. ovata*, in products such as Metamucil. As with other foods that provide bulk, it has been shown to reduce cholesterol levels. Applied externally, the plant stimulates and cleanses the skin and encourages wounds to heal faster. Plantain has also been used to dye wool a dull gold or camel color.

Use fresh plantain leaves for poultices. Chew the fresh root for toothache. You can make the leaves into a tincture, tea, or pills. For urinary tract problems, they are often mixed with dandelion root, and for infection, they are mixed with uva ursi. To make an herbal combination for coughs and bronchial congestion, mix plantain with elecampane and mullein. Add fresh leaves and fresh or dried roots to any all-purpose skin salve.

Part used: Leaves, root, seed

Preservation: Harvest fresh leaves any time. You can preserve the properties of plantain leaves and roots in lotions and salves. Dig the root in fall and use fresh or dried. Harvest seeds when ripe, shake and blow off the shaft, and grind them.

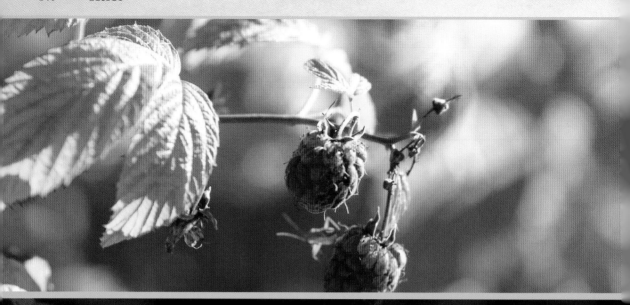

Raspberry

Perennial

Botanical Name: *Rubus idaeus*

Family: Rosaceae

Height: 4 ft.

Spread: 3 ft.

Description: Native to North America and Europe, this shrubby, thorny plant, also known as hindberry and bramble, quickly spread around the world. You'll find raspberry thickets along the edges of woods and in untended fields. The raspberry plant produces a prickly stem. Its flowers are white and appear in the spring and summer of its second year. Berries ripen in June and July. Each fruit is composed of lots of little fruits, or drupelets, which give it its familiar shape. The plant produces erect shoots or canes that, in time, flop over and reproduce. Raspberry leaves are pale green above, gray-white beneath, and serrated with a rounded base.

Ease of care: Easy

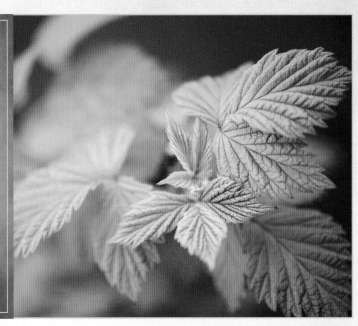

Raspberry leaves are thought to tone uterine muscles and, thus, have long been used by pregnant women to prevent miscarriage and reduce labor pains. They can be used throughout pregnancy. They relieve menstrual cramps if taken as a tonic over a period of time. Raspberry leaves are also good for women with uterine problems such as fibroids, endometriosis, or excessive menstrual bleeding.

Cultivation: The plant prefers full sun in loose, rich, well-drained soil, with manure or compost.

Propagation: Divide roots or plant 1/2-inch cuttings in a few inches of soil. But be careful that your raspberry bushes do not take over your garden. Once rooted, the plant is prolific, sending up new shoots with frequency.

Uses: Long revered for its healing properties, raspberry is an astringent, stimulant, and tonic. Seventeenth-century English herbalist Nicholas Culpepper recommended raspberry for a number of ailments, including "fevers, ulcers, putrid sores of the mouth and secret parts . . . spitting blood . . . stones of the kidney . . . and too much flowing of women's courses." American Indians used raspberry as a treatment for wounds. And contemporary herbalists prescribe raspberry for diarrhea, nausea, vomiting, and morning sickness.

The fruit is a tonic and may be good for the blood. Fresh raspberries can have a mild laxative effect, but a tea from the leaves is a cure for diarrhea and dysentery. Fresh or frozen raspberries have many uses in the kitchen.

The leaves of raspberry make a tasty hot or iced tea. During pregnancy, mix them with other gentle herbs such as lemon grass or chamomile for some variety. To prevent miscarriage, use equal parts raspberry leaf, false unicorn root, and cramp bark; drink 2 to 3 cups a day. If using tincture of raspberry, take 1/4 to 1/2 teaspoon (1 to 2 droppers full) a day, as needed. Use raspberry tea externally as a wash for sores, ulcers, and raw skin surfaces. Eat the fruit fresh, or freeze or preserve in vinegar or liquor.

Part used: Fruit, leaves

Preservation: Harvest berries in summer. Harvest leaves any time, but the best time is before the plant bears fruit; use fresh or dried.

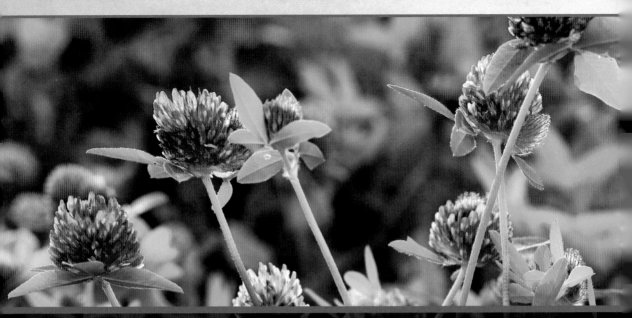

Red Clover

Perennial

Botanical Name: *Trifolium pratense*

Family: Fabaceae (Leguminosae)

Height: To 2 ft.

Spread: 8 in.; invasive

Description: This wide-ranging legume produces leaves in groups of three and fragrant red or purple ball-shaped flowers. Like its relatives, beans and peas, red clover adds nitrogen to the soil. Sufficient nitrogen is important to produce healthy plants. As a result, red clover is a popular winter and early spring cover crop to enrich the soil, but because it is a tenacious perennial that spreads by means of runners, it must be well chopped before you replant the garden. You'll find it growing in fields and vacant lots. The plant is widely cultivated.

Ease of care: Easy

Cultivation: Red clover thrives in moist, well-drained soil with full sun.

Propagation: Sow seeds in the spring or fall.

Uses: Red clover, a favorite of honey bees, is one of the world's oldest agricultural crops. This ubiquitous field flower has been used as a medicine for millennia, revered by Greeks, Romans, and Celts. But it's in the last 100 years that red clover has gained prominence as the source of a possible cancer treatment. Researchers have isolated several antitumor compounds such as biochanin A in red clover, which they think may help prevent cancer. The herb also contains antioxidants and a form of vitamin E. There is some evidence that it helps prevent breast tumors.

Some of red clover's constituents are thought to stimulate the immune system. Another constituent, coumarin, has blood-thinning properties. Its hormone-mimicking effect makes red clover a potential treatment for some types of infertility and symptoms of menopause. A diuretic, sedative, and anti-inflammatory herb, red clover has been recommended for the skin conditions eczema and psoriasis. It also has some anti-bacterial properties.

You may pick flowers and add them to salads throughout the summer. Tiny florets are a delightful addition to iced tea. Eat red clover's nutritious leaves cooked since they are not digestible raw.

Take 1 to 2 teaspoons (4 to 8 droppers full) of tincture up to three times a day.

Part used: Flowers, leaves

Preservation: Gather leaves and flowers in early summer when tops are in bloom.

Precautions: Avoid red clover if you're pregnant or have a history of bleeding easily. Also, because it is a blood thinner, avoid it just before surgery.

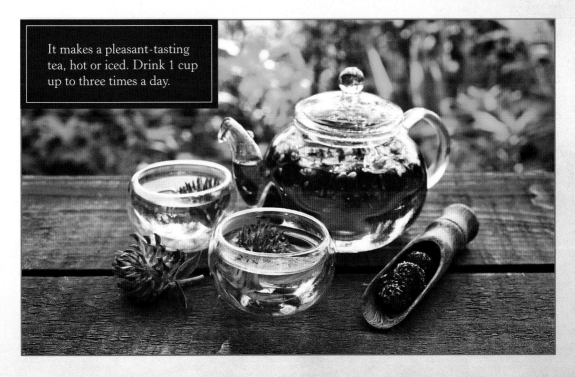

It makes a pleasant-tasting tea, hot or iced. Drink 1 cup up to three times a day.

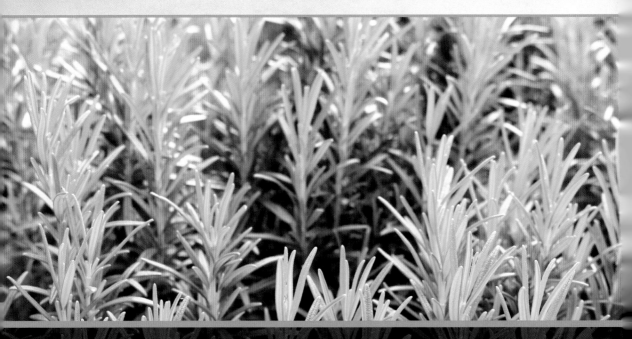

Rosemary

Perennial

Botanical Name: *Rosmarinus officinalis*

Family: Lamiaceae (Labiatae)

Height: 4–6 ft.

Spread: 2–4 ft.

Description: Rosemary makes a stunning addition to any garden. An attractive, spreading evergreen, its gray-green, needle-shaped leaves may be pruned to form a low hedge. A low-growing variety of rosemary provides a wonderful ground cover. The herb produces pale blue flowers from December through spring. Rosemary is found on hills along the Mediterranean, in Portugal, and in northwestern Spain. The herb is cultivated widely elsewhere.

Ease of care: Moderate

Cultivation: Rosemary likes sandy, alkaline soil and full sun but will grow in partial sun. Grow rosemary as a potted plant in cold climates, or protect it from winter winds.

Propagation: Sow seed; take cuttings or layer in spring.

Uses: Before the advent of refrigeration, cooks wrapped meat in rosemary leaves to preserve it. The herb's strong piney aroma has prevented commercial use as a preservative, but efforts are underway to create a preservative without the scent. Modern studies show that rosemary has potent antioxidant properties. It is an astringent, expectorant, and diaphoretic (induces sweating). It promotes digestion and stimulates the activity of the liver and gallbladder to aid both in digestion of fats and the detoxification of the body. It also inhibits formation of kidney stones. The herb has been prescribed to treat muscle spasms. Rosemary oil helps reduce the pain of rheumatism when used as a liniment. An antiseptic, it can be applied to eczema and wounds. It strengthens blood vessels and improves circulation, so it is useful to treat varicose veins and other problems related to poor circulation. For this reason, it can also relieve some headaches. A foot bath containing rosemary is good for swollen ankles and feet that tend to be numb or cold often—both signs of poor circulation. It makes a good gargle for sore throats, gum problems, and canker sores. New studies indicate that compounds in rosemary may help to prevent cancer.

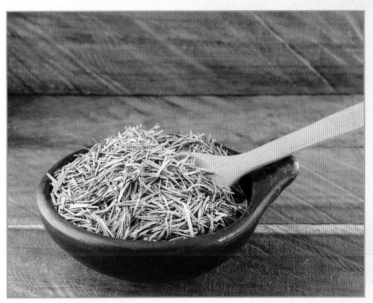

In the kitchen, rosemary's pungent taste—something like mint and ginger—complements poultry, fish, lamb, beef, veal, pork, game, cheese, and eggs, as well as many vegetables, including potatoes, tomatoes, spinach, peas, and mushrooms. Rosemary essential oil is found in soaps, creams, lotions, and perfumes. The oil and herb are added to cosmetics to improve skin tone. The herb makes a fragrant, refreshing bath additive and hair rinse. It stimulates the scalp and helps control dandruff. And dried branches make good arrangements and wreaths. Also add rosemary to lotions, cream, and salves for its skin-healing properties. It is often combined with lavender in aromatherapy products to sweeten its pungent aroma. To improve circulation, use a rosemary liniment, or add a few drops of the essential oil to a bath or to a pan of water for soaking feet or hands.

Part used: Leaves; branches in decorations

Preservation: Pick rosemary leaves when needed and use fresh. Hang-dry stems or freeze 3 to 4-inch growth tips.

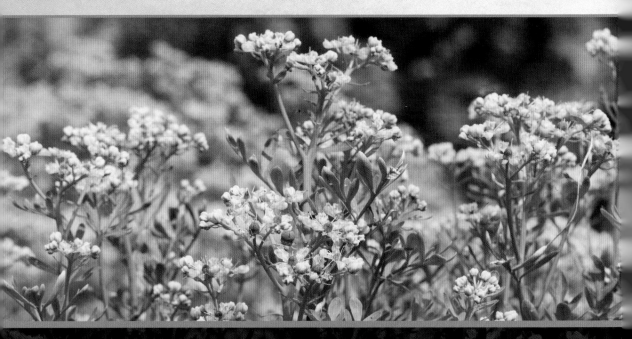

Rue

Perennial

Botanical Name: *Ruta graveolens*

Family: Rutaceae

Height: 3 ft.

Spread: 2 ft.

Description: Rue produces blue-green, teardrop-shaped leaves in clusters. It is an attractive and unusual plant to use as a focal point in a garden design, producing yellow to yellow-green flowers from June through August. Rue is native to southern Europe. The plant is no longer found in the wild but is cultivated widely in Europe and America.

Ease of care: Easy

Cultivation: Rue prefers full or partial sun in poor, sandy, alkaline soil in a location protected from the wind. It may be grown easily as a potted plant. Some gardeners advise that you don't plant rue near basil, sage, or cabbage, but rue is said to enhance growth of figs and roses.

Propagation: Sow seed outdoors in spring, or start indoors a few weeks before the last frost and transplant once the soil has warmed. Take cuttings in midsummer.

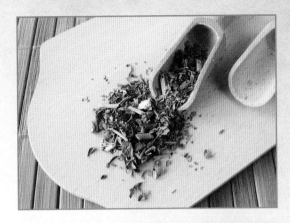

Uses: The Greeks believed that rue cured indigestion, improved eyesight, and treated insect bites. Today, rue is more popular as a medicine in several countries other than the United States. The exception is the Latino community in the United States. They use *Ruta* to relieve menstrual cramps and to regulate menstruation. Throughout Latin America, people use rue tea to treat colds and rue compresses applied to the chest to treat congestion. Rue is also used as a liniment to relieve the pain of rheumatoid arthritis and sore muscles. In traditional Chinese medicine, rue is used to decrease the inflammation of sprains, strains, and bites. Rue contains rutin, which strengthens fragile blood vessels, so the herb helps diminish varicose veins and reduces bruising when used internally or topically. Rue eardrops decrease the pain and inflammation of an earache.

Taken internally, rue relaxes muscles and nervous indigestion and improves circulation in the digestive tract. People in the Middle East use it to kill intestinal parasites, and in India, they say it improves mental clarity, which is possible because of its action on circulation.

Although it is bitter, minute amounts are used to flavor some baked goods. The Italians use rue as a bitter digestive, eating small amounts with other bitter greens and using it in a liqueur, *grappa con ruta.*

Rue tea is extremely bitter—and potent—so it is best combined with other herbs. Take no more than 1 cup of tea or 1/4 teaspoon (1 dropper full) of tincture a day of pure rue. For a liniment, combine it with rosemary and heating herbs such as cayenne and peppermint in an alcohol base. Apply the tincture directly to bruises, varicose veins, and any inflammation.

Dried rue seed heads add interest and texture to arrangements.

Part used: Leaves, seed heads

Preservation: Pick leaves just before the flowers open, and hang them to dry. Collect the seed heads when they begin to dry.

Precautions: Use rue internally with extreme caution: It may cause gastrointestinal pains. Large amounts cause vomiting, mental confusion, and convulsions. And in rare cases, exposure to sunlight after ingesting rue causes severe sunburn. The entire plant is covered in glands that produce an essential oil, which irritates the skin of some people. If you are one of these people, wear gloves when handling rue. It is a uterine stimulant, so do not use during pregnancy.

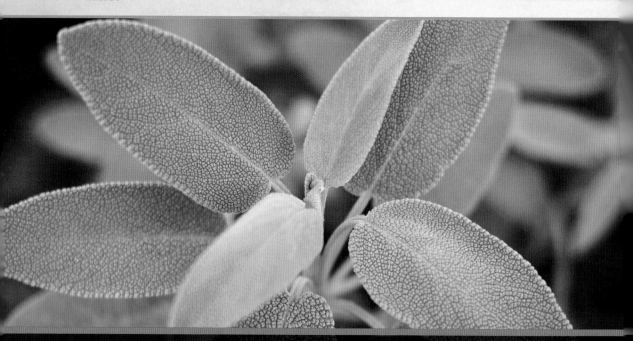

Sage

Perennial

Botanical Name: *Salvia officinalis*

Family: Lamiaceae (Labiatae)

Height: 3 ft.

Spread: 2 ft.

Description: Sage produces long, oval, gray-green, slightly textured leaves; it comes in variegated and purple-leaved varieties. Sage is a good edging plant, attractive in any garden. In June, the herb produces whorls of pink, purple, blue, or white flowers. Sage is native to the Mediterranean. A hardy plant, it has become naturalized elsewhere and is cultivated as far north as Canada.

Ease of care: Easy

Cultivation: Sage prefers full sun in a well-drained, sandy, alkaline soil. Protect it from the wind. Sage is said to enhance growth of cabbages, carrots, strawberries, and tomatoes, but some gardeners recommend that you keep it away from onions.

Propagation: Sow seed, take cuttings, divide, or layer in spring.

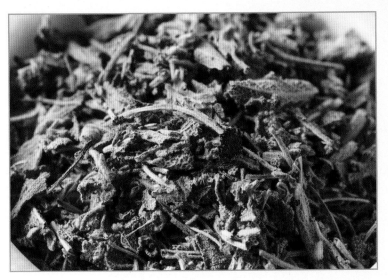

Uses: You may associate sage with Thanksgiving. The herb is often used to flavor poultry dressings. The Arabs associated sage with immortality, and the Greeks considered it an herb that promotes wisdom. Appropriately enough, a constituent in sage was recently discovered to inhibit an enzyme that produces memory loss and plays a role in Alzheimer disease. However, it's unlikely that use of the herb alone will benefit these conditions. Sage's essential oils have antiseptic properties, and the tannins are astringent. It has been used for centuries as a gargle for sore throat and inflamed gums. The herb is useful in treating mouth sores, cuts, and bruises. Sweating is decreased about two hours after ingesting sage; in fact, it is used in some deodorants and a German antiperspirant. It is also use-ful to prevent hot flashes, and it has some estrogenic properties. It decreases mother's milk so is useful while weaning children. It decreases saliva flow in the mouth and has successfully been used by people who have overactive salivary glands. It is a strong antioxidant and may prove useful against cell degeneration in the body. As a hair conditioner, a sage infusion reduces overactive glands in the scalp, which are sometimes responsible for causing dandruff. It also gives gloss to dark hair.

Sage's sharp, almost camphorlike taste complements salads, egg dishes, soups, breads, marinades, sausage, beef, pork, veal, fish, lamb, duck, goose, and a variety of vegetables, including tomatoes, asparagus, beans, and onions.

Sage is sometimes found in perfumes and cosmetics. Dried leaves on the branches make a good ornamental that complements arrangements and wreaths. Sage dyes wool shades of yellow or green-gray.

Use sage in food or tea; however, as tea, sage is best mixed with other herbs that are not as pungent-tasting, such as mint.

Part used: Leaves

Preservation: Harvest sage and use fresh as needed. Hang leaves to dry or lay on a screen, or freeze.

Precautions: In large amounts, thujone, a constituent of sage, may cause a variety of symptoms, culminating in convulsions, but it is safe in the small amounts found in sage leaves.

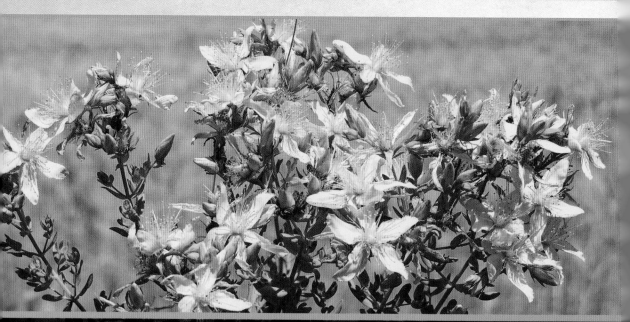

St. John's Wort

Perennial

Botanical Name: *Hypericum perforatum*

Family: Hypericaceae

Height: To 3 ft.

Spread: 1 ft.

Description: The bright yellow flowers of this erect herb appear from June to July. Green leaves are small and oblong and appear to have "pores" when held up to the light. Native to Europe, St. John's wort has become naturalized throughout North America in woods and meadows. St. John's wort received its name perhaps because it blooms around June 24, the day celebrated as the birthday of Christ's cousin, John the Baptist. The herb exudes a reddish oil from its glands when a leaf is crushed.

Ease of care: Easy

Cultivation: St. John's wort is a wild herb that may be transplanted to a garden. A hardy herb, it will grow in most soils.

Propagation: Sow seed in spring.

Uses: St. John's wort has been used as a medicine for centuries. Early European and Slavic herbals mention it. It has long been used as an anti-inflammatory for bruises, varicose veins, hemorrhoids, strains, sprains, and contusions. It is used internally and topically (in tincture, oil, or salve form) for these conditions. The plant, especially its flowers, is high in flavonoid compounds that reduce inflammation.

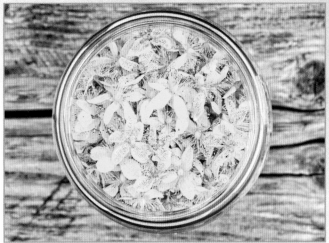

Studies show that St. John's wort relieves anxiety and is an antidepressant. Some researchers believe that one of its constituents, hypericin, interferes with the body's production of a depression-related chemical called monoamine oxidase (MAO). In one study, it relieved depression in menopausal women in four to six weeks.

The herb has also been used to treat skin problems, urinary conditions such as bed-wetting, painful nerve conditions such as carpal tunnel syndrome, and symptoms of nerve destruction. The tannin and oil in the plant have antibacterial properties. Scientists investigating the potential of one of its constituents as a treatment for AIDS discovered it also fights viral infection. It is also effective against flu. The National Cancer Institute has conducted several preliminary studies showing that constituents in St. John's wort also may have potential as a cancer-fighting drug. The herb dyes wool shades of yellow and red.

Take 1/2 to 1 teaspoon (2 to 4 droppers full) of tincture up to three times a day. To make St. John's wort oil, soak puréed leaves and flowers in olive oil. Keep in a warm place for 4 to 6 days. Strain and apply topically. St. John's wort must be used fresh to acquire its active ingredients, so make your own oil or tincture, or purchase only products made from the fresh plant. You can take St. John's wort pills, but be sure they are made from either freeze-dried herbs or a dried extract since the herb loses most of its medicinal properties when air-dried.

Part used: Leaves, flowers

Preservation: Gather leaves and flowers after the plant has bloomed. Tincture or infuse in oil when fresh—the herb loses much of its medicinal properties when dried. Store oil in a dark container; it should keep for two years.

Precautions: After consuming large quantities of the herb, cattle develop severe sunburn and become disoriented; however, there are no documented reports of humans having this reaction. Recent testing among AIDS patients showed that St. John's wort is nontoxic. Avoid St. John's wort if you take an MAO inhibitor drug.

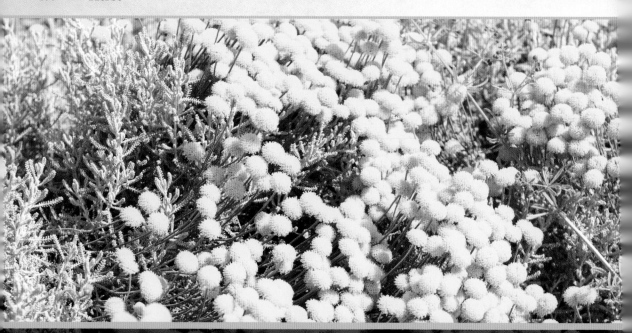

Santolina

Perennial

Botanical Name: *Santolina chamaecyparissus*

Family: Asteraceae (Compositae)

Height: 1–2 ft.

Spread: 1 ft.

Description: This spreading evergreen produces light silver-gray, cottony leaves with an interesting knobby look. The herb makes a great edging or low hedge and was once popular in knot gardens. Santolina is a member of the daisy family, and its bright yellow flowers appear in June and July. Santolina, also known as grey santolina, is native to the Mediterranean region and cultivated widely.

Ease of care: Easy

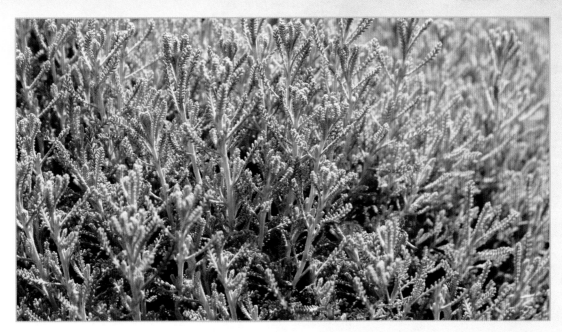

Cultivation: Santolina likes full sun and average, sandy, preferably alkaline soil. In severely cold climates, protect your plants, or grow them in pots and bring them inside when temperatures drop.

Propagation: Sow seed in the spring; cut, divide, or layer in early summer.

Uses: Santolina's most important modern use is as a garden ornamental. Drought resistant and attractive as a ground cover, it is popular for landscaping in southern California and other dry regions of the Southwest. It is often planted as a fire break. A dwarf santolina (*S. chamaecyparissus* 'Nana') makes a low, tight-growing ground cover. Other members of the family are the cultivar "Plumosus" with its feathery leaves, and a green santolina (*S. virens*).

Once used to expel parasitic worms, this astringent herb is rarely prescribed for medicinal purposes in the West, but it is an antiseptic for bacterial and fungal skin infections. It can be rubbed into sore muscles as a liniment. Small quantities of this herb taken internally act as a digestive bitter that stimulates appetite and digestion. Santolina has a musky fragrance that enhances potpourri and sachets. The essential oil is sometimes used in perfumes. Fresh branches are used to make herbal wreaths, although you must work with them when they are still fresh; they become quite brittle when they dry. The plant dyes wool shades of gold and yellow. Speaking of wool, the strong scent of the leaves also repels wool moths. Place a sachet containing the leaves in among sweaters and blankets in drawers, closets, or storage boxes.

Ingesting large amounts of santolina can cause digestive upsets, rather than cure them.

Infuse in vegetable oil for a liniment. You can take a few tablespoons of tea to aid digestion, but be forewarned—it is very bitter!

Part used: Leaves; branches for decoration

Preservation: Harvest leaves and branches in late summer. Hang-dry.

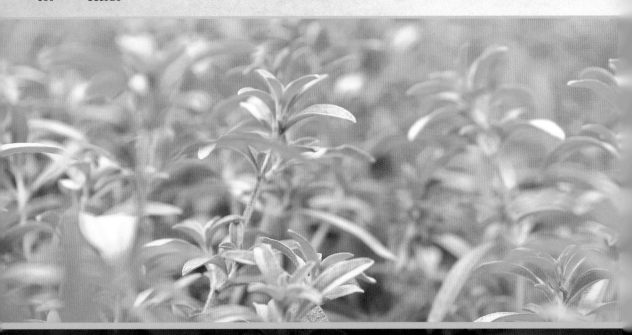

Savory, Summer

Annual

Botanical Name: *Satureja hortensis*

Family: Lamiaceae (Labiatae)

Height: 1–1 1/2 ft.

Spread: 8–12 in.

Description: This attractive annual has soft, flat, gray-green, narrow leaves. The plant has a light, airy appearance. Winter savory (*S. montana*) is a hardy perennial. Summer savory is tastier but has a shorter growing season than winter savory: It flowers from midsummer to the first frost. Both savories are native to the Mediterranean region; summer savory has become naturalized in North America, Asia, and Africa.

Ease of care: Easy

Cultivation: Summer savory likes full sun in a light, average, sandy soil. The herb does not like to be transplanted. It grows easily in containers.

Propagation: Sow seed in spring after the soil is warm.

Uses: The Romans believed savory was sacred to satyrs, mythical man-goats who were said to roam the forests. The Romans also planted it near beehives to increase honey production. They used savory to flavor vinegars and introduced the herb to England, where the Saxons adopted and named it for its spicy taste. Winter savory was said to curb sexual appetite; summer savory, to increase it. Guess which variety was most popular? Summer savory has antiseptic and astringent properties, so it has been used to treat diarrhea and mild sore throats. Like many culinary herbs, it aids digestion, stimulates appetite, and relieves a minor upset stomach and eliminates gas—probably one reason it is so popular to flavor bean dishes. It also kills several types of intestinal worms. If you are unfamiliar with the herb, try using it in recipes that call for parsley or chervil. It is often considered a lighter substitute for sage or thyme.

To receive savory's medicinal properties, use it in foods. If you find the essential oil, use it to make antiseptic skin salves.

Part used: Leaves

Preservation: Harvest leaves when the plant begins to flower; hang or dry on screens.

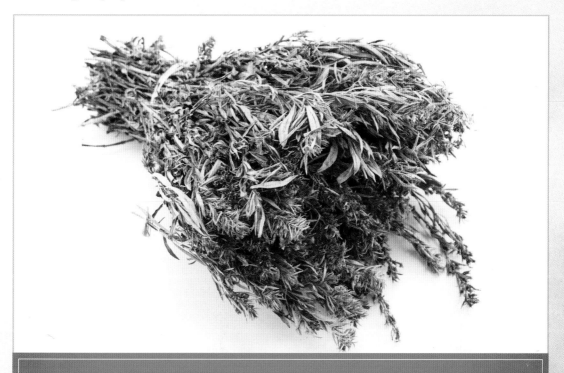

In the kitchen, summer savory's flavor, reminiscent of thyme, brings out the best in butters, vinegars, beans, soups, eggs, peas, eggplant, asparagus, onions, and cabbage. It is one of the flavorings in salami and other commercial foods.

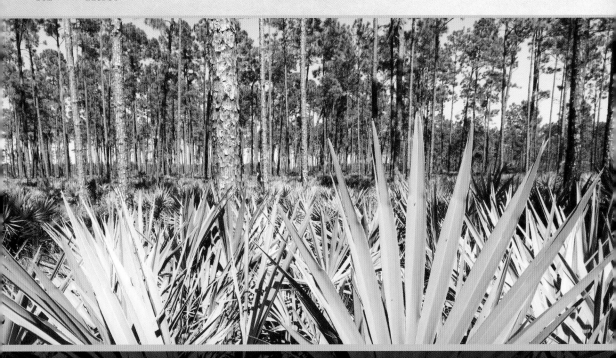

Saw Palmetto

Perennial

Botanical Name: *Serenoa repens*

Family: Palmaceae

Height: To 6 ft.

Spread: Sprawls

Description: Saw palmetto is a low, shrubby plant with a creeping trunk. It produces palmlike, deeply divided leaves. Olive-shaped berries are dark purple to black and grow in bunches, ripening from October to December. The herb is found in dense stands along the Atlantic coasts of Georgia and Florida.

Ease of care: Easy

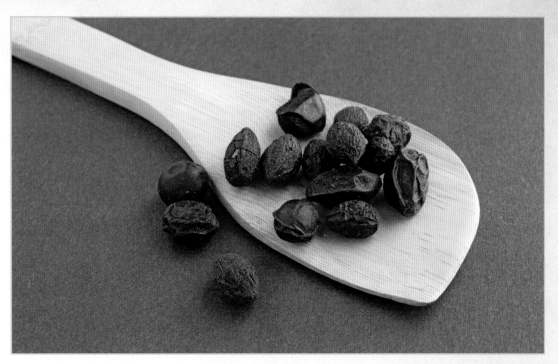

Cultivation: Saw palmetto is a wild plant that thrives in swampy, well-drained soils. It needs hot weather and temperatures that do not dip below freezing to survive.

Propagation: Transplant plants. It can also be grown from seed, but this is more difficult.

Uses: Saw palmetto has long been considered an aphrodisiac, sexual rejuvenator, and treatment for impotence. The action of saw palmetto has been well studied, and the herb is popular for treating prostate enlargement. In one study, participants experienced significant improvement in prostate enlargement in only 45 days, with almost no side effects, and certainly none of the serious side effects seen with the drugs normally prescribed. Saw palmetto is recommended for weakening of urinary organs and resulting incontinence.

Saw palmetto also has been touted as a steroid substitute for athletes who wish to increase muscle mass, although documentation is scanty. Herbalists agree, however, that saw palmetto may benefit cases of tissue wasting, weakness, and debility. It was prescribed by Eclectic physicians in the early 19th century for frail people or those who were weak from chronic illness to make them stronger. This may be because saw palmetto improves digestion and absorption of nutrients. The herb is a diuretic, expectorant, and tonic, making it useful for treating colds, asthma, and bronchitis.

Drink up to 2 cups of tea a day. Take 1/4 to 1 teaspoon (1 to 4 droppers full) of tincture up to twice a day. Saw palmetto is often combined in preparations with other prostate herbs, such as nettle root and the African herb pygeum.

Part used: Berries

Preservation: Gather the fruit after berries turn black. Dry or tincture.

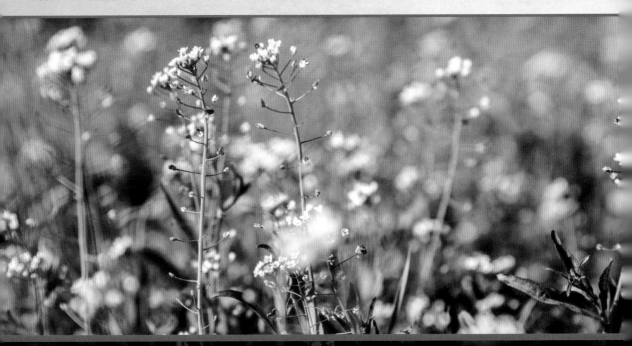

Shepherd's Purse

Annual or Biennial

Botanical Name: *Capsella bursa-pastoris*

Family: Cruciferae

Height: 1 ft.

Spread: 6 in.; may become invasive

Description: This herb's name alludes to the shape of its fruits, which resemble the purses that Europeans once hung from their belts. Smooth, slightly hairy stems arise from a basal rosette of leaves. The herb produces white flowers throughout the year, followed by triangular-shaped fruits. Shepherd's purse is found frequently in gravelly, sandy, or loamy soil. It grows just about everywhere, including Greenland, where it was introduced by Vikings more than a thousand years ago.

Ease of care: Easy

Cultivation: Shepherd's purse is not often cultivated, perhaps because it grows so readily as a garden weed; you can also find it readily in the wild. The herb tolerates most soils but prefers well-drained, sandy loam and full sun to partial shade. The plant can become invasive.

Propagation: Shepherd's purse grows easily from seeds sown in spring.

Uses: The Greeks and Romans used the seeds of shepherd's purse as a laxative. By the 16th century, the herb was prescribed to stop bleeding and eliminate blood in urine. Colonists introduced shepherd's purse to America, where it quickly became a common weed.

Shepherd's purse contains substances that hasten coagulation of blood—thus it has long been prescribed for treating excessive menstrual flow. During World War I, wounded soldiers were given shepherd's purse tea. The herb also may benefit those with ulcers, colitis, and Crohn disease. Used topically, shepherd's purse heals lacerations and other skin injuries. Some herbalists have prescribed it for treating eczema and skin rashes. The herb's peppery-tasting young leaves may be added to soups and stews or eaten like spinach.

For excessive menstrual bleeding, take a few days to a week before the period and during the period. Drink up to 1 cup, several times a day. The tea is bitter tasting, so you may want to mix it with another herb. Take 1/2 teaspoon (2 droppers full) of tincture twice a day.

Part used: Leaves and the flower tops

Preservation: Harvest leaves and flower tops as flowers open. Dry or tincture. The fresh plant is more potent than the dried plant.

Precautions: Because shepherd's purse constricts blood vessels and appears to induce clotting, people with a history of hypertension, heart disease, or stroke should avoid it.

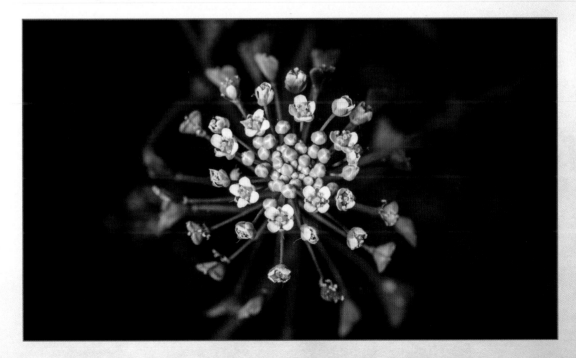

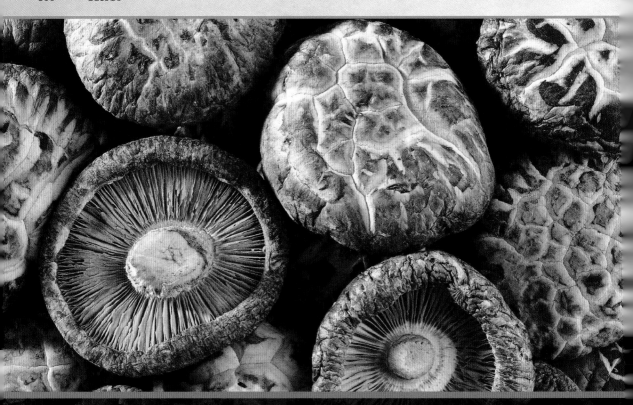

Shiitake Mushroom

Annual

Botanical Name: *Lentinus edodes*

Family: Tricholomataceae

Height: To 6 in.

Spread: To 6 in.

Description: The shiitake mushroom is a fungus that grows on dead tree trunks in the wild.

Ease of care: Moderate

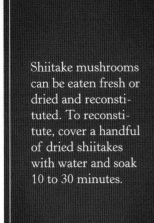

Shiitake mushrooms can be eaten fresh or dried and reconstituted. To reconstitute, cover a handful of dried shiitakes with water and soak 10 to 30 minutes.

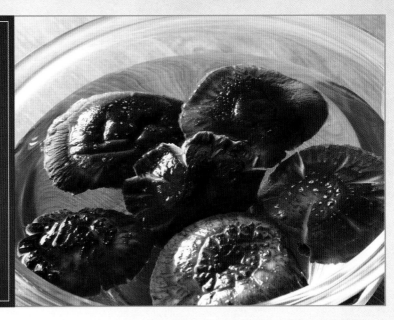

Cultivation: Shiitakes and other mushrooms are cultivated commercially and found in the wild. Years ago, few people would have tried to grow their own shiitake mushrooms, but the popularity of the mushroom due to its flavor and medicinal qualities has led to a great interest among growers. The traditional method of growing shiitakes is to use hardwood logs as a host in which to place the spawn—the material used to propagate mushrooms. Shiitake mushrooms require moisture and darkness to grow. When you purchase a kit to grow these (or any) mushrooms, you will receive detailed instructions on how to grow them.

Propagation: Mushrooms reproduce by spores.

Uses: Shiitake mushrooms have long been a staple of Chinese cuisine. Now research has found that lentinan, a chemical in shiitake mushrooms, slows the growth of cancerous tumors in animals. Scientists hope that lentinan may one day be used to enhance the human immune system and help people fight off cancer and infections.

In China and Japan, shiitake mushrooms have been used for hundreds of years as a medicine to lower blood cholesterol as well as to fight cancer. Shiitake mushrooms also contain cortinelin, a strong antibacterial agent, which kills a wide range of disease-causing germs. A sulfide compound extracted from shiitake mushrooms has also been found to have antibiotic properties. Shiitakes have been used to treat depressed immune-system disorders, including AIDS.

Use in foods such as soups, stews, and noodle dishes. Chinese physicians recommend eating 2 to 4 ounces of shiitake mushrooms two to three times a week to prevent cancer. Shiitake is also available in pills or as a tincture. Take the amounts suggested on the manufacturer's package.

Shiitake mushrooms are a nutritious food source, packed with protein and full of vitamins B1, B2, B12, niacin, and pantothenic acid.

Part used: Mushroom caps

Preservation: Dry for teas and tinctures.

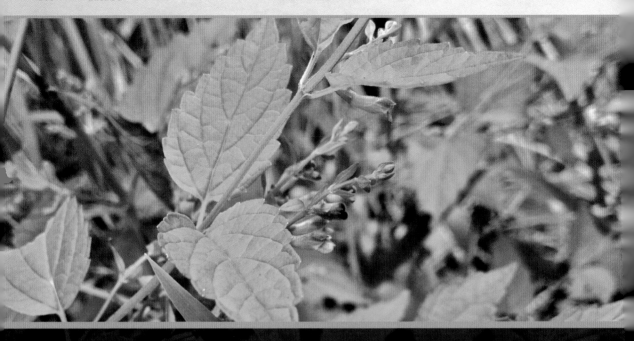

Skullcap

Perennial

Botanical Name: *Scutellaria lateriflora*

Family: Lamiaceae (Labiatae)

Height: 1–2 ft.

Spread: 8 in., spreading

Description: Skullcap is a slender, branching, square-stemmed plant with opposite, serrated leaves. Its blue flowers, which have two "lips," resemble the skullcaps worn in medieval times, hence, the herb's name. Several species of skullcap grow in Europe and Asia. Also known as mad dog weed and Virginia skullcap, the herb is found throughout the United States and southern Canada.

Ease of care: Moderate

Cultivation: Skullcap prefers well-drained, moist soil and partial shade. Once rooted, the herb requires little care.

Propagation: Sow seeds or divide roots in early spring. Thin seedlings to 6 inches.

Uses: Skullcap received its common name, mad dog weed, in the 18th century, when the herb was widely prescribed as a cure for rabies, although no scientific evidence supports its use for that disease. The herb is a sedative often recommended for treating insomnia, nervousness, nervous twitches, and anxiety. Russian researchers have found that skullcap helps stabilize stress-related heart disease. Herbalists have also employed skullcap to treat symptoms of premenstrual syndrome (PMS). Skullcap has been found to have anti-inflammatory properties. The herb inhibits release of acetylcholine and histamine, two substances released by cells that cause inflammation and symptoms of allergic reactions. Japanese studies indicate that skullcap increases levels of HDL (high-density lipoprotein, or "good" cholesterol). And Chinese researchers report that the Chinese species, *S. baicalensis*, is useful in treating hepatitis, improving liver function, reducing swelling, and increasing appetite. It is also a strong immune system herb.

Take skullcap as a tea, a tincture, or in pills. The taste is slightly bitter, so most people mix it with peppermint or chamomile when they drink it as a tea. In formulas to ease nervous system problems, it is mixed with herbs such as valerian, passion flower, and chamomile. Take up to 2 cups of tea or 1/2 teaspoon (2 droppers full) of tincture a day.

Part used: Leaves

Preservation: Gather leaves after flowers bloom in summer; dry or tincture.

Precautions: Used in moderation, skullcap is safe. Large amounts of tincture may cause confusion, giddiness, or convulsions.

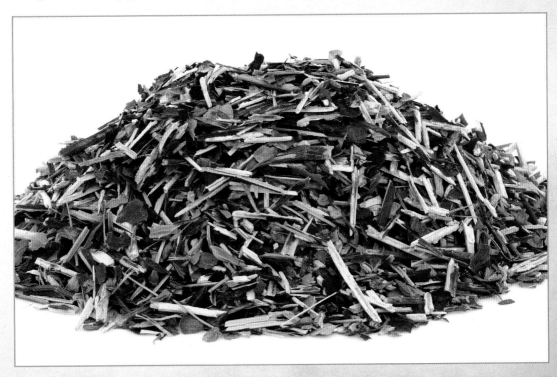

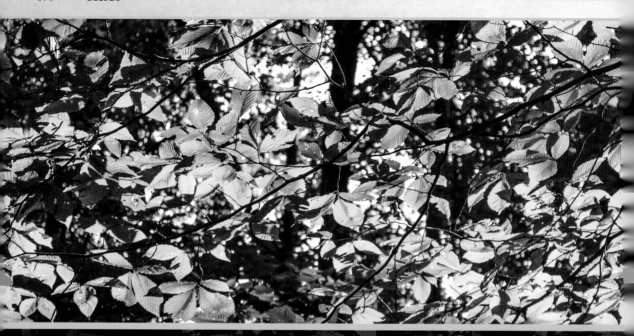

Slippery Elm

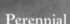

Perennial

Botanical Name: *Ulmus rubra* (previously *U. fulva*)

Family: Ulmaceae

Height: To 60 ft.

Spread: 25 ft.

Description: The trunk bark of this stately tree is brown, but branch bark is whitish. Slippery elm leaves are broad, rough, hairy, and toothed. The tree is native to North America from southern Canada to Florida. In the 18th and 19th centuries, American forests were covered with elms, but most succumbed to Dutch elm disease. Today slippery elm is found in far fewer numbers in moist woodlands and along streams.

Ease of care: Easy

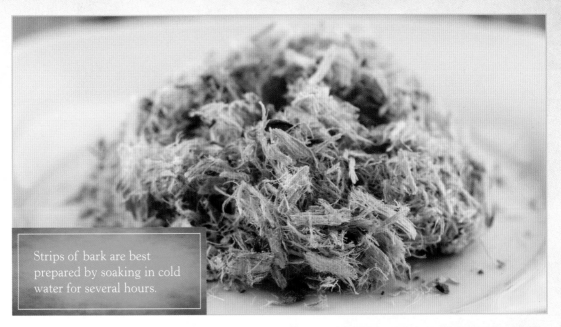

Strips of bark are best prepared by soaking in cold water for several hours.

Cultivation: Slippery elm prefers average soil and requires sun and moisture. You can grow it in a yard, provided you have enough space.

Propagation: Purchase seedlings to plant.

Uses: American colonists learned from Indians how to employ the herb as a food and medicine. In the days before refrigerators, Americans wrapped foods in slippery elm to slow spoilage: The powdered bark contains cells that expand into a spongy mass to form a protective covering. They also used moistened slippery elm powder to form bandages, make casts for broken bones, coat pills, and make a nourishing gruel for invalids. In the last century, you would have been hard-pressed to find a home in America that did not contain slippery elm lozenges.

Slippery elm is used to treat sore throats, coughs, colds, and gastrointestinal disorders—in a word, anything that needs to be soothed. Mucilage, the most abundant constituent in the bark, has a moistening, soothing action. The tannins are astringent.

This combination makes slippery elm ideal for soothing inflammations, reducing swelling, and healing damaged tissues.

The powder is a healing food. Stir slippery elm powder into oatmeal or applesauce for an oatmeal-like gruel that soothes an inflamed stomach or ulcer. It is often recommended as a restorative herb for people who suffer from prolonged flu, stomach upset, chronic indigestion, and malnutrition stemming from these conditions.

Stir 2 to 3 tablespoons of the powdered bark in juice, fruit, oatmeal, or other foods. You may also mix slippery elm powder with hot water, bananas, and applesauce. In treating sore throat and coughs, slippery elm is most effective made into lozenges or syrup. Today, due to the increasing scarcity of slippery elm, herbalists often use alternative herbs such as comfrey for topical use and marshmallow for internal use.

Part used: Inner bark

Preservation: Powder the bark.

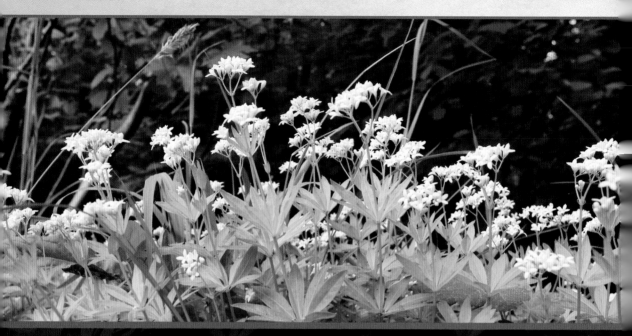

Sweet Woodruff

Perennial

Botanical Name: *Galium odoratum* (previously *Asperula odoratum*)

Family: Rubiaceae

Height: 6–8 in.

Spread: 6 in.

Description: Sweet woodruff produces small, knife-shaped leaves that circle in tiers around the stemlike wheel spokes. This rich green perennial spreads by means of underground stems to make a lovely ground cover. Its white, funnel-shaped flowers appear in May and June. Native to Europe, North Africa, and Asia, the herb is often found deep in forests.

Ease of care: Easy

Cultivation: Sweet woodruff insists on average, moist soil in woodland shade.

Propagation: Sow seed in fall to sprout in spring; divide after the plant flowers, allowing several months for the roots to re-establish themselves before the first frost.

Uses: Herbalists consider sweet woodruff a diuretic, diaphoretic, antispasmodic, and light sedative. It is especially useful to treat nervous indigestion. The herb has been used historically to treat kidney stones, nervousness, and wounds. It is also an anticoagulant, thereby reducing the risk of blood clots. Sweet woodruff has been used to flavor Scandinavian cordials, and it imparts a sort of vanilla-like bouquet to white wine. It is the flavoring in Europe's traditional May wine and other alcoholic beverages. (The FDA approves its use for alcoholic beverages.) The herb is used in potpourri and perfumes; its scent, described as like that of new-mown hay, is due to coumarin, which is also found in hay and clover. Branches dye wool tan; roots yield a red dye.

Sweet woodruff can be made into tea but is a more popular remedy infused in wine. To make May wine, add a handful of the chopped fresh or dried herbs to a liter of white wine. Let sit four weeks, then strain and serve. Apply mashed, fresh leaves to wounds.

Part used: Leaves

Preservation: Pick fresh sweet woodruff and use as needed. The scent increases as it dries. Hang to dry or lay on screens.

Precautions: Very large doses of sweet woodruff may cause vomiting and dizziness. Test animals suffered liver damage, among other effects, when fed coumarin, a constituent of sweet woodruff, but you would have to eat massive amounts daily to reach an equivalent amount.

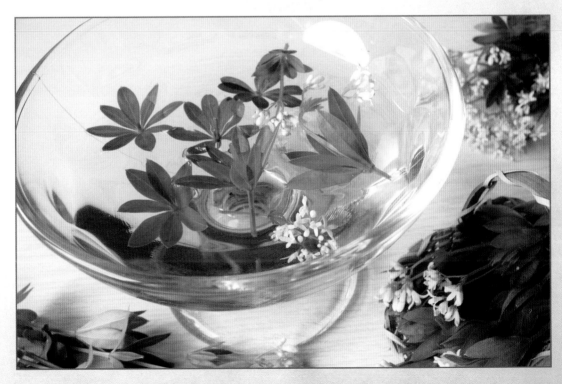

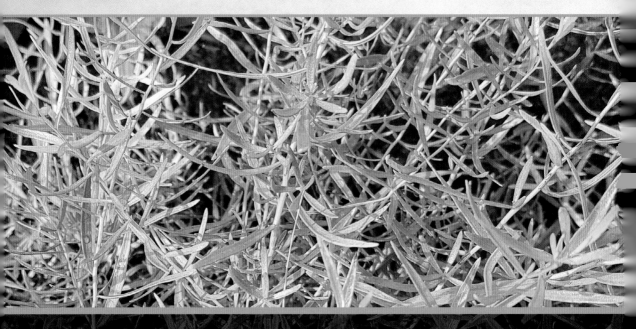

Tarragon, French

Perennial

Botanical Name: *Artemisia dracunculus*

Family: Asteraceae (Compositae)

Height: 2 ft.

Spread: 1 ft.

Description: This perennial has long, narrow, pointed leaves, but its flowers rarely appear. Be sure to get the French rather than the Russian variety of tarragon. The Russian variety looks much the same but has somewhat narrower, lighter green leaves, and it flowers and produces seed. But Russian tarragon has less of the sweetly aromatic flavor of its French cousin. Test the plant by crushing, smelling, and tasting a few leaves. Tarragon is probably native to the Caspian Sea area and possibly Siberia and Europe. It is cultivated in Europe, Asia, and the United States.

Ease of care: Moderate

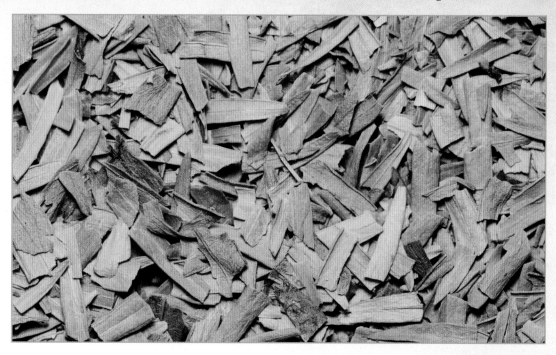

Cultivation: Tarragon prefers full sun to partial shade in a sandy, average, well-drained alkaline soil. It may also be grown successfully as a potted plant. Cut tarragon back in the fall or early spring. Protect it with mulch during winter. Tarragon is said to enhance the growth of most companion vegetables.

Propagation: Since it produces no seeds, buy your first plant, then take cuttings in summer and fall; divide or layer in early spring.

Uses: Thomas Jefferson was one of the first Americans to grow this lovely and useful plant. Tarragon stimulates appetite, relieves gas and colic, and makes a good local anesthetic for toothaches. Tarragon has antifungal and antioxidant properties and has been used to preserve foods. It's also found in perfumes, soaps, cosmetics, condiments, and liqueurs. One of the French *fines herbes*, tarragon has a strong flavor that may overpower foods, so use it sparingly in salads and sauces, including remoulade, tartar, and bearnaise sauces. Tarragon enhances fish, pork, beef, lamb, game, poultry, patés, rice, barley, vinegars, mayonnaise, and butter. It also goes well with a number of vegetables, including potatoes, tomatoes, carrots, onions, beets, asparagus, mushrooms, cauliflower, and broccoli.

Use tarragon in cooking. Chew the fresh leaves to relieve a toothache.

Part used: Leaves

Preservation: Pick leaves at any time for fresh use. Cut the stems and hang to dry. Don't dry tarragon too long or it will lose its flavor. Store immediately in an airtight container. You can also capture tarragon's flavor in vinegar or oil.

Precautions: For culinary use, tarragon is considered safe. Although the plant contains estragole, which produces tumors in mice, it has not been associated with human cancer.

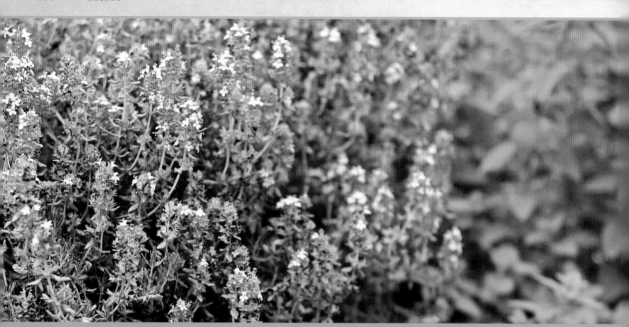

Thyme

Perennial

Botanical Name: *Thymus vulgaris*

Family: Lamiaceae (Labiatae)

Height: 10–12 in.

Spread: 1–1 1/2 ft.

Description: These tiny-leaved, wide-spreading perennials make a good inexpensive ground cover that can be clipped and mowed regularly. Thyme's profuse lilac to pink blooms appear in June and July and are especially attractive to bees. Native to the western Mediterranean region, thyme is cultivated widely. There are many species and varieties of thyme with self-descriptive names, including woolly thyme, silver thyme, lemon thyme, and golden thyme.

Ease of care: Easy

Cultivation: Thyme does well in full sun in poor to average, well-drained soil. Trim it back each spring to encourage abundant new growth. It also may be grown as a potted plant. Some gardeners believe that thyme enhances growth of eggplant, potatoes, and tomatoes. It is said to repel cabbage worms and whiteflies.

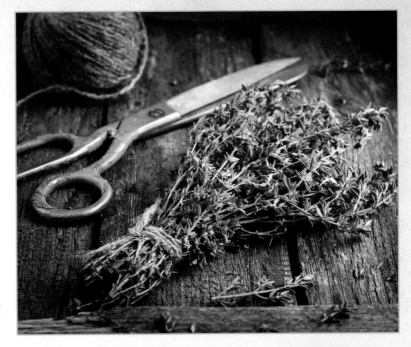

Propagation: Sow seed or divide in spring or fall; take cuttings or layer in early summer.

Uses: You may have noticed thyme's distinctive flavor in cough medicines. Thymol, a prime constituent, is found in a number of them. Thymol is also used commercially to make colognes, aftershaves, lotions, soaps, detergents, and cosmetics. Thyme was used as an antiseptic to treat wounds as recently as World War I. In fact, it is one of the most potent antiseptics of all the herbs. Thymol is found in mouthwashes and gargles for sore throats and mouth and gum infections. It is one of the main ingredients in Listerine, along with compounds from eucalyptus and peppermint. This commercial mouthwash was found to cause 34 percent less gum inflammation than other brands and decrease plaque formation on the teeth. Vapor balms, used to rub on the chest to relieve congestion, also contain thymol. Thyme destroys fungal infections. Its antispasmodic qualities make it useful for treating asthma, whooping cough, stomach cramps, gas, colic, and headache. It also reduces compounds in the body that produce menstrual cramps. Thyme preparations increase circulation in the area where applied.

One of the French *fines herbes*, thyme complements salads, veal, lamb, beef, poultry, fish, stuffing, patés, sausage, stews, soups, bread, butters, mayonnaise, vinegars, mustard, eggs, cheese, and many vegetables, including tomatoes, onions, eggplant, leeks, mushrooms, asparagus, and green beans.

Thyme is used medicinally in foods. Sometimes it is used in tinctures for digestive problems, but more often, it is in liniments, salves, skin antiseptics, cough syrup and drops, mouthwashes, and vapor balms.

Part used: Leaves

Preservation: Harvest leaves any time for fresh use. Pick before and during flowering, and hang-dry.

Precautions: In moderate amounts, thyme causes no problems, but use the essential oil carefully: It can burn the skin.

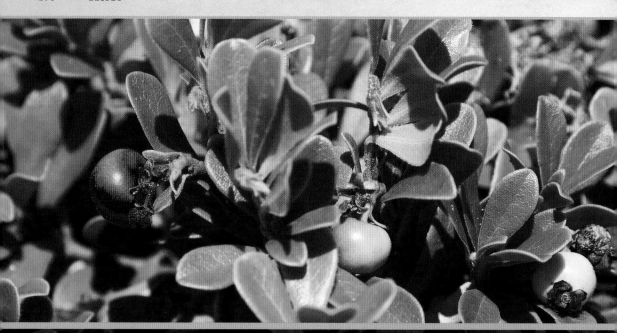

Uva Ursi

Perennial

Botanical Name: *Arctostaphylos uva ursi*

Family: Ericaceae

Height: 6 in.

Spread: 3 in.

Description: Uva ursi's pink-red berries are a favorite food of bears, hence the herb's common name, bearberry. Because uva ursi leaves were often used as tobacco, the plant also is known as *kinnikinnick*, a Native American word that means smoking mixture. Uva ursi is a delicate ground cover with fibrous roots and leathery, oblong leaves. The herb produces white, red-tinged flowers in April and May. Uva ursi is found throughout the northern hemisphere, especially in dry, rocky areas.

Ease of care: Easy

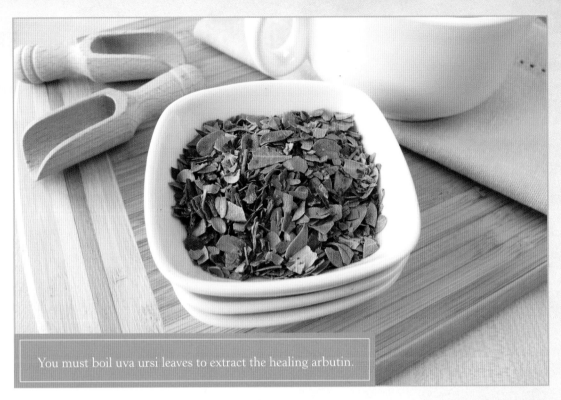

You must boil uva ursi leaves to extract the healing arbutin.

Cultivation: Uva ursi can sometimes be purchased at nurseries as a ground cover. Sow seeds in the fall or spring. The herb likes peaty soil and full sun. Uva ursi needs little care, except for watering. The herb is generally free of pests and disease.

Propagation: Sow seeds in the spring; take cuttings or layer in spring.

Uses: Uva ursi leaves contain up to 40 percent tannic acid, enough to make them once useful in tanning leather. Tannins and the glycoside arbutin give uva ursi its astringent and antiseptic properties.

Herbalists suggest uva ursi primarily to treat bladder infections. Uva ursi is particularly indicated for illnesses caused by *E. coli*. It works particularly well in the alkaline environment this bacteria produces. Externally, the herb has been used to treat sprains, swellings, and sore muscles.

Drink up to 3 cups of uva ursi tea a day. For a tea low in tannic acid, infuse the herb in cold water for 12 to 24 hours. Take 1/4 to 1 teaspoon (1 to 4 droppers full) of tincture up to three times a day. Mix uva ursi with milder urinary herbs such as marshmallow and fennel seed.

Uva ursi dyes wool shades of camel to green.

Part used: Leaves

Preservation: Gather leaves in spring or early summer. Tannin levels increase in fall, so gather only young leaves. Dry for infusions, or tincture.

Precautions: Because uva ursi may stimulate the uterus, don't take it if you're pregnant. Also don't use it if you have an active kidney infection since it will be too irritating.

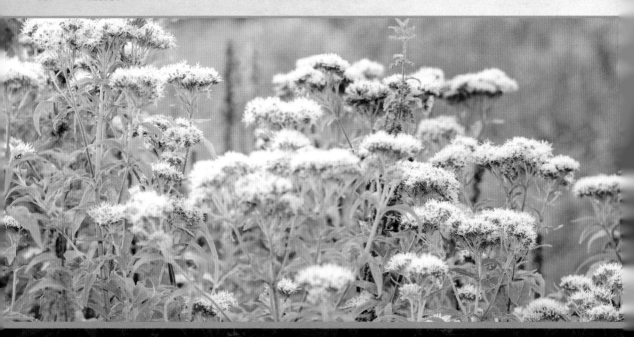

Valerian

Perennial

Botanical Name: *Valeriana officinalis*

Family: Valerianaceae

Height: 3–5 ft., in flower

Spread: 1 ft.

Description: There are some 200 species of valerian, a plant with an erect, hollow, hairy stem that produces four to eight pairs of dark green leaves. Held on tall, thin stalks, valerian flowers are small and pink-tinged and appear in June through July. Various medicinal species of the herb are native to Europe and western Asia and grow wild in North America. There are also several native American species. You may find valerian in grasslands, damp meadows, and along streams.

Ease of care: Easy

Cultivation: Valerian prefers rich, moist, humusy soil and full sun to partial shade.

Propagation: Divide roots in spring or fall. Seeds germinate poorly. Sow them in a cold frame in April and transplant in May. Divide valerian every three years to prevent overcrowding.

Uses: Ask most people what the smell of valerian reminds them of and they're likely to say old socks. Nonetheless, cats go wild over valerian and so do rats. Lore has it, in fact, that the Pied Piper used valerian to rid Hameln of rodents. In ancient times, valerian was widely used as a treatment for epilepsy. Today valerian finds its chief value in soothing anxiety and promoting sleep. Clinical studies have identified constituents in valerian known as valepo-triates, which appear to affect the central nervous system but produce few, if any, side effects. Several studies show that valerian shortens the time needed to fall asleep and improves quality of sleep. Unlike commonly used sedatives, valerian does not cause a drugged or hung-over sensation or affect dream recall in most people. In one study, it even calmed hyperactive children.

The relaxing action of valerian also makes it useful for treatment of muscle cramps, menstrual cramps, and high blood pressure. Valerian relaxes vein and artery walls and is especially indicated for blood pressure elevations caused by stress and worry. Valerian is recommended for tension headaches as well as heart palpitations.

Valerian mildly stimulates the intestines, can help dispel gas and cramps in the digestive tract, and is weakly antimicrobial, particularly to bacteria. More than a hundred soothing valerian preparations are sold in Germany. Valerian improves stomach function and relieves gas and painful bowel spasms. The herb has been used commercially to flavor tobacco and some beverages.

Valerian has a disagreeable taste, so mix it with other herbs such as peppermint if you drink it as tea. Take a cup of tea or 2 capsules of the powdered root an hour before bed. Or take 1/2 to 1 teaspoon (2 to 4 droppers full) of tincture up to three times a day. It is often combined with other sedative herbs such as skullcap, chamomile, and lemon balm.

Part used: Root

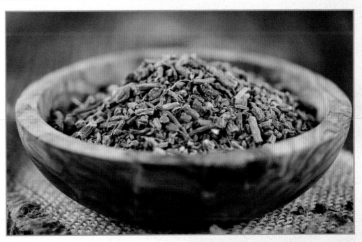

Preservation: Gather roots in fall or spring, before shoots appear, and dry.

Precautions: Valerian occasionally has the opposite effect of that intended, stimulating instead of sedating. Reducing the dosage usually alleviates the problem. Valerian may cause headaches, dizziness, and heart palpitations when taken in large doses. Don't take valerian if you're pregnant.

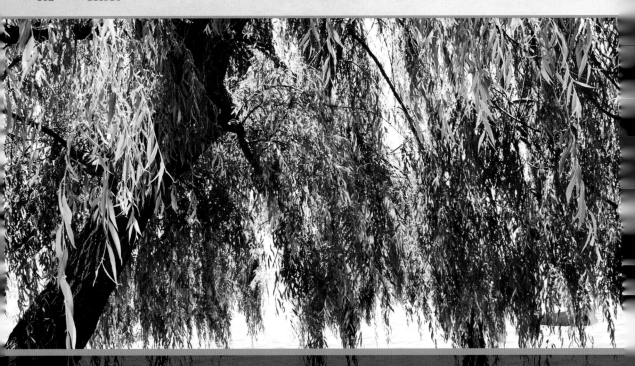

Willow

Perennial

Botanical Name: *Salix spp.*

Family: Salicaceae

Height: 35–75 ft.

Spread: To 5 ft.

Description: The ubiquitous willow is found throughout temperate regions of the Northern hemisphere. Its long leaves on flexible branches are narrow and lance-shaped, lending the tree a graceful appearance. Willows have tiny flowers in cylindrical catkins and blossom in midspring. The tree's bark is rough and grayish brown.

Ease of care: Moderate

Cultivation: Often found along river banks, willow likes soggy soil but will grow well in any moist garden bed. The tree prefers full sun.

Propagation: Willow cuttings root easily. In moist soil, root young, leafless branches several feet long. In spring, take hardwood cuttings 9 to 12 inches long and root in water. Even leafy summer cuttings will root. The problem is that rooted cuttings are sometimes difficult to transplant. When you succeed in getting new plants to grow, stand back: Cuttings grow quickly and must be pruned back diligently. Don't worry about over-pruning. The tree will come back bushier than ever.

Uses: Although their long billowing branches bring to mind "weeping," willows were considered a symbol of joy by the ancient Egyptians, who prized the trees that grew along the banks of the Nile. And well they should have. This attractive shade tree is also a potent healer.

The various species of willow contain salicin, from which salicylic acid, the main ingredient of aspirin, is derived, and herbalists often recommend the plant to relieve pain. The Chinese have been putting it to this purpose since 500 BC. It's also a useful herb for women with painful periods. Willow contains enough salicylate to suppress chemicals known as prostaglandins, one cause of painful menstrual cramps.

Willow is also used to treat fever, headache, hay fever, neuralgia, and inflammation of joints. Take willow as tincture, tea, or pills. The tea is bitter so most people prefer to get their medicinal dose of willow in tincture or pill form. Pills are sold both as capsules and tablets and can be used in place of aspirin. Take up to 4 cups of tea, 1 teaspoon (4 droppers full) of tincture, or 6 pills a day.

Willow's lovely foliage enhances decorative arrangements. Willow wood is extremely supple and has long been used to make baskets.

Part used: Bark, shoots, wood

Preservation: Harvest bark and wood any time. Gather shoots in the spring. Use willow fresh or dried.

Precautions: In animal studies, aspirin has been associated with increased risk of birth defects, thus, avoid willow if you are pregnant. Also, the use of aspirin in children has been linked to Reye syndrome, a rare but potentially fatal disease. Although willow has not been associated with Reye syndrome, it's still best not to give willow to children with colds, flu, or chicken pox.

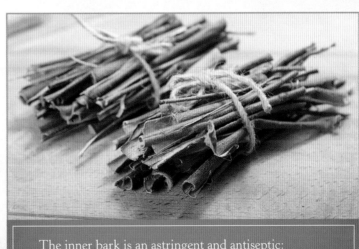

The inner bark is an astringent and antiseptic: Decoctions of white willow bark are valued in facial lotions and baths for their astringent properties.

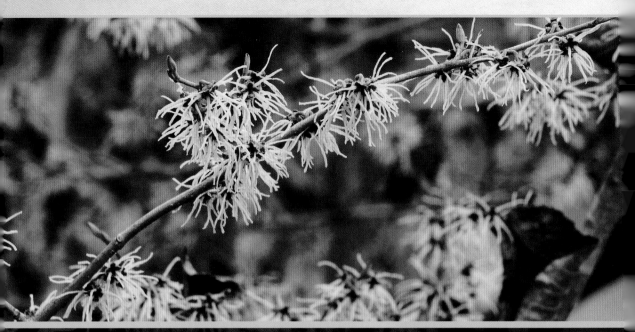

Witch Hazel

Perennial

Botanical Name: *Hamamelis virginiana*

Family: Hamamelidaceae

Height: 8–15 ft.

Spread: 15 ft.

Description: Witch hazel is a small, deciduous tree, with twisting stems and long, forked branches. The herb's smooth bark may be gray or brown, its leaves oval. Bright-yellow flowers are threadlike and appear in September and October. Some species bloom in winter. The plant is indigenous to North America, from Quebec south to Florida and west to Minnesota and Texas. You're likely to encounter witch hazel in moist, light woods or along rocky streams.

Ease of care: Moderate

Cultivation: Witch hazel prefers moist, rich, neutral to acid soil, and full sun to partial shade.

Propagation: To germinate seeds, expose them to temperatures of 40 degrees Fahrenheit for three months. You can also propagate witch hazel by taking cuttings or by layering.

Uses: Witch hazel has long been prized as an astringent cosmetic and medicinal herb. Its leaves, twigs, and bark contain tannic and gallic acids and essential oils. Witch hazel dries weeping, raw tissues. A cloth soaked in strong witch hazel tea and applied to the skin reduces the swelling and pain of hemorrhoids, bruises, wounds, and sprains and promotes speedy healing. It can also tighten and soothe aching varicose veins and reduce inflammation associated with blood clots (phlebitis) in the legs.

Witch hazel lotions are useful on rough, swollen hands. And the herb is a popular skin cleanser and body lotion; it is also effective in treating insect bites, sunburns, and poison oak and ivy rashes and is an ingredient in aftershaves. The herb is also used as a mouthwash, gargle, and douche.

Drink a cup of witch hazel tea up to three times a day. Take up to 1/2 teaspoon (2 droppers full) of tincture, two to six times a day. Limit use to a few weeks.

To make witch hazel lotion, place twigs and bark in a blender with enough vodka to cover. Chop as fine as possible, and transfer to a glass jar. Shake the mixture vigorously once a day and strain after two weeks. Blend 1 ounce of witch hazel liquid with 1/2 ounce aloe vera gel and 1/2 ounce vitamin E oil. Store in a tightly stoppered bottle.

A tincture made from witch hazel, goldenseal (or Oregon grape root), and calendula and applied to the outer ear is useful to treat swimmer's ear. This same combination in an infusion makes an effective douche for vaginal infections. A gargle of 8 ounces of witch hazel tea and a couple drops of the essential oils of myrrh and clove bud reduces the pain of a sore throat, or, as a mouth rinse, treats swollen, infected gums. Also use this as a pain- and inflammation-relieving gum rub for teething babies. A tea made from witch hazel, chamomile, mint, and thyme is effective for diarrhea.

Part used: Leaves, twigs, bark

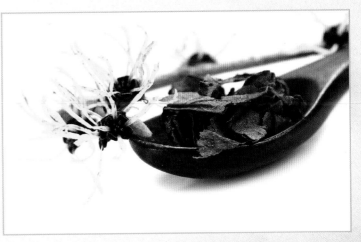

Preservation: Gather leaves, twigs, and bark in early fall before the tree flowers; dry or tincture.

Precautions: The tannins in witch hazel may produce nausea if consumed in large quantities. Pay attention to the label of any witch hazel prepation you purchase. While you can ingest the tincture made with grain alcohol, many preparations are made from the poisonous rubbing (isopropyl) alcohol.

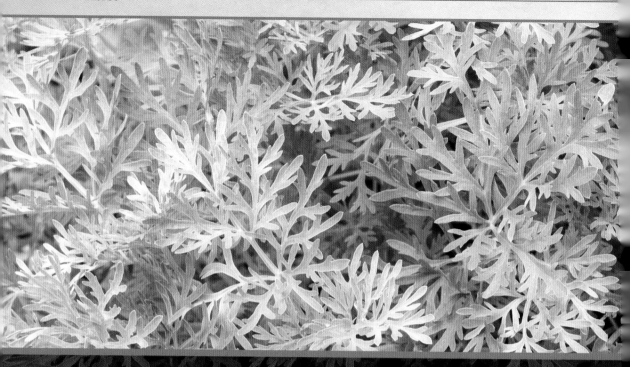

Wormwood

Perennial

Botanical Name: *Artemisia absinthium*

Family: Asteraceae (Compositae)

Height: 3–4 ft.

Spread: 2 ft.

Description: Wormwood produces handsome, fine, silver-green leaves. The plant flowers in July and August and is at the height of its glory in autumn. It is a hardy herb, unharmed by frost. Wormwood is native to the Mediterranean region and has become naturalized throughout the temperate world. It is cultivated widely.

Ease of care: Easy

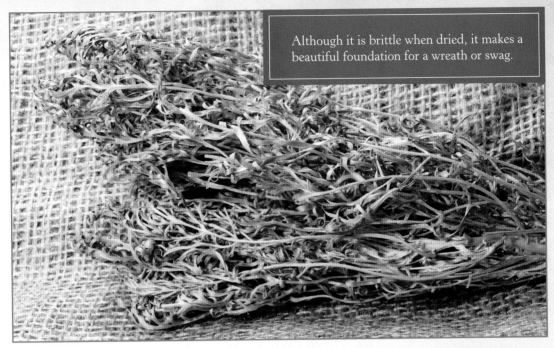

Although it is brittle when dried, it makes a beautiful foundation for a wreath or swag.

Cultivation: Like the other popular species of Artemisia, southernwood (*A. abrotanum*), wormwood likes full sun in almost any kind of soil, as long as it's alkaline. Add lime if soil is naturally acidic.

Propagation: Sow seed or take cuttings in summer; divide in spring or fall.

Uses: Wormwood is steeped in mystique. It is said to have grown up in the trail left by the serpent as it slithered from the Garden of Eden. The herb is a prime ingredient of an alcoholic drink called absinthe, which is illegal in most countries, including the United States. Wormwood got its name because it expels intestinal worms. The plant also is an antiseptic, antispasmodic, and carminative, and it increases bile production. It has been used to treat fever, colds, jaundice, and gallstones.

Compresses soaked in the tea are said to be good for irritations, bruises, and sprains. Wormwood oil has been used as a liniment to relieve the pain of rheumatism, neuralgia, and arthritis. The plant is also an antifungal and antibacterial, and new research indicates that compounds in one of the species of wormwood, *A. annua*, could be a cure for malaria. Wormwood is also a flea and moth repellant.

Part used: Leaves; branches in arrangements

Preservation: Harvest leaves after the plant flowers. Hang to dry. Store in airtight containers.

Precautions: In large doses, wormwood's active constituent, thujone, is a convulsant, poison, and narcotic. The herb is not very water-soluble, but tinctures are high in thujone, so don't use tinctures internally. Topical use is generally considered safe, but wormwood may cause dermatitis in some people. Do not use wormwood internally for more than a couple days unless you are under the supervision of a physician or qualified herbalist and not at all if you are pregnant.

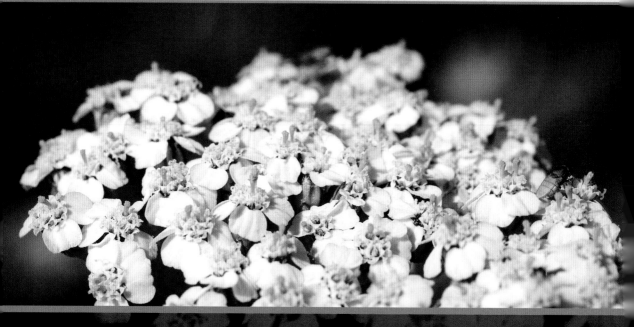

Yarrow

Perennial

Botanical Name: *Achillea millefolium*

Family: Asteraceae (Compositae)

Height: To 3 ft.

Spread: To 1 ft.

Description: Yarrow's Latin name means "a thousand leaves," a reference to the herb's fine, feathery foliage. Erect and covered with silky "hairs," yarrow produces white flower heads from June through September. The herb is native to Europe but has become naturalized throughout North America. You'll find yarrow growing along roads and in fields and waste places.

Ease of care: Easy

Cultivation: Yarrow likes full sun and well-drained soil. The herb will adapt to almost any type of garden except those with soggy soil. Creeping species of yarrow, which may be mowed, will rot unless the soil is well drained. Occasionally, yarrow falls prey to powdery mildew, rust, or stem rot. Yarrow may benefit companion plants by attracting helpful insects, such as wasps and lady bugs.

Propagation: Sow seed in the spring; divide in spring or fall.

Uses: In the epic *Iliad*, Homer reports that legendary warrior Achilles used yarrow leaves to treat the wounds of his fallen comrades. Studies show that yarrow is a fine herb indeed for accelerating healing of cuts and bruises. The Greeks used the herb to stop hemorrhages. Gerard's famous herbal cited yarrow's benefits in 1597. And after colonists brought the plant to America, Indians used it to treat bleeding, wounds, infections, headaches, indigestion, and sore throat.

Clinical studies have supported the long-standing use of yarrow to cleanse wounds and make blood clot faster. Yarrow treats bleeding stomach ulcers, heavy menstrual periods, and bleeding from the bowels. An essential oil known as azulene is responsible for yarrow's ability to reduce inflammation. Traditional Chinese medicine credits yarrow with the ability to nurture the spleen, liver, kidney, and bladder. Several studies have shown that yarrow improves uterine tone and reduces uterine spasms in animals. Apigenin and flavonoid constituents are credited with yarrow's antispasmodic properties.

The herb also contains salicylic acid, aspirin's main constituent, making it useful for relieving pain. Chewing the leaves or root is an old toothache remedy. Yarrow fights bacteria and dries up congestion in sinus and

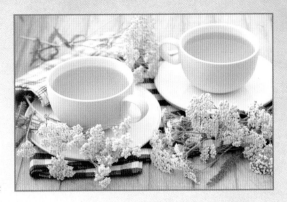

other respiratory infections and allergies. The plant has long been a standby herb for promoting sweating to bring down fevers in cases of colds and influenza. It also relieves bladder infections.

Because of its astringent and cleansing properties, yarrow is sometimes added to skin lotions. Flowers and stalks dry well, making attractive decorations. The flowers dye wool shades of yellow to olive.

Chew fresh yarrow root for relief of toothache. Press mashed fresh leaves or powdered dried leaves or flower tops over cuts to stop bleeding. Soak a cloth in yarrow tea and apply this compress to wounds and bruises. Take 1/2 to 2 teaspoons (2 to 8 droppers full) of tincture or several cups of tea up to three times a day. A popular tea to reduce fever is made with equal parts of yarrow, elderberry flowers, and peppermint. Drink it hot and it reduces a fever; the cold tea is a diuretic.

Part used: Flowers, leaves, roots

Preservation: Gather flowers in late spring or early summer, when the plant is in full bloom. Dig roots in fall. Dry for teas or preserve in tinctures.

Precautions: Some people are sensitive to yarrow. The most common indicators of sensitivity are sneezing, headache, or nausea.

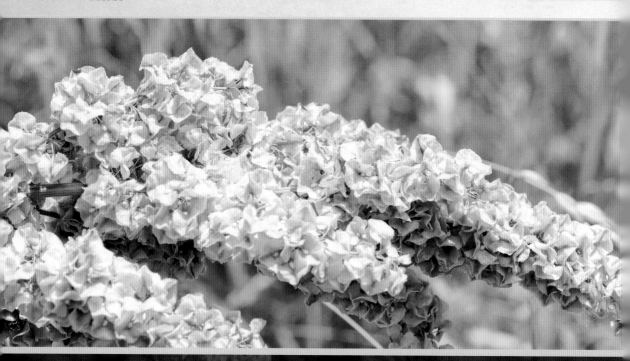

Yellow Dock

Perennial

Botanical Name: *Rumex crispus*

Family: Polygonaceae

Height: To 3 ft.

Spread: 1 ft.

Description: Yellow dock produces a yellow taproot, leaves that taper to a point, and whorls of greenish flowers that appear on tall stems in midsummer. The herb is native to Eurasia and grows as a weed throughout temperate and subtropical regions.

Ease of care: Easy

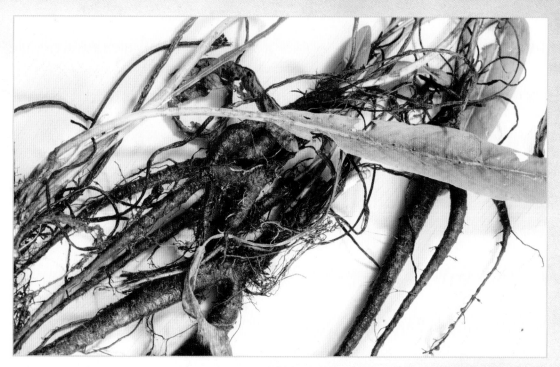

Cultivation: Yellow dock is a wild plant that likes poor to average soil in weedy places.

Propagation: Plants grow from seed in spring.

Uses: Yellow dock root stimulates intestinal secretions and promotes bile flow, which aids fat digestion and has a light laxative action. The root is also used to treat anemia and can dramatically increase iron levels in the blood in only a few weeks. Long considered a blood purifier, yellow dock may also be effective in treating a number of conditions that stem from liver dysfunction, including skin eruptions, headaches, and unhealthy hair and nails. An astringent and tonic, yellow dock has been used to treat ringworm, laryngitis, and gingivitis.

Steam or sauté very young leaves as you would greens. The tall flower stalks are used in dried flower arrangements and are prized by flower arrangers because they retain their attractive rusty-red color when dried.

You can drink up to 3 to 4 cups a day of yellow dock tea. However, yellow dock is bitter, so add herbs such as peppermint or lemon balm to improve the flavor. Take up to 1/2 teaspoon (2 droppers full) of the tinc-ture a day.

Part used: Root, leaves; flower stalks for dried arrangements

Preservation: Gather roots in the fall; dry or tincture. Gather young leaves in early spring and eat fresh.

Precautions: Although it is unlikely that anyone would want to do so, eating several bowls of dock salad could cause gas, cramping, and diarrhea. The leaves contain oxalic acid, which may contribute to some types of kidney stones. The root should be avoided by people with a history of gall-bladder attacks.

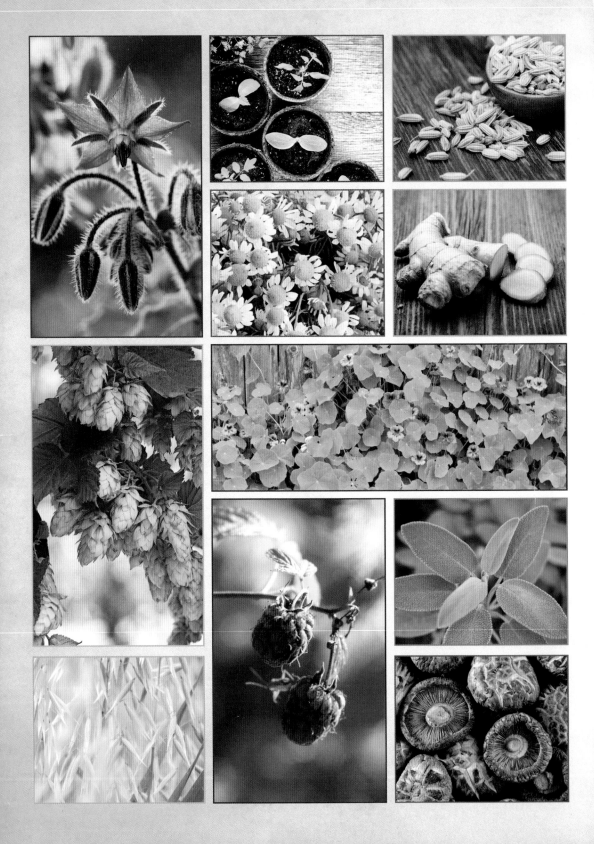